"With a rare combination of clinical wisdom and testable scientific clarity, therapists at every level of experience will find in these pages a compassionate guide for the real work of change, one that may also help move the field beyond brand loyalty and toward process-based knowledge."

Steven C. Hayes, *PhD, Foundation Professor of Psychology Emeritus, University of Nevada, Reno, and originator of acceptance and commitment therapy*

"Brilliant."

Marvin R. Goldfried, *PhD, Distinguished Professor of Psychology (ret.), Stony Brook University*

"In this highly engaging and unifying guide, Dr. Jeffery Smith distills decades of wisdom into clear principles that demystify the therapeutic process. Bridging across schools of thought, he offers therapists from beginner to experienced practitioner both confidence and practical direction. A must read for anyone seeking to understand how psychotherapy truly fosters healing and growth."

Dilip Jeste, *MD, past president of the American Psychiatric Association, president elect, World Federation for Psychotherapy*

"The future of psychotherapy depends upon people like Jeffery Smith. This is an important book."

Mark Solms, *PhD, Professor of Neurophysiology, University of Cape Town*

"Few have been as dedicated as Dr. Smith to the work of bringing together rival schools of psychotherapy. This invaluable book will help therapists of all stripes understand more clearly what they are doing and how it works as they also find common ground."

Eric M. Plakun, *MD, past Medical Director/CEO, Austen Riggs Center, founder of the American Psychiatric Association Psychotherapy Caucus*

How Psychotherapy Works

How Psychotherapy Works synthesizes recent science to provide an accessible, practical, and clinically relevant understanding of the infrastructure underlying the hundreds of therapies in current use. In joining the best of modern neuroscience with a warm-hearted understanding of human troubles, the book guides beginning and experienced therapists to better therapy through clarity about what is happening now and what to do next.

Both groundbreaking and paradigmatic, the book extends modern concepts of memory reconsolidation and thinking fast and slow to bring to light the nonconscious world where problematic patterns are frozen in time, waiting for empathic connection with a therapist. The final section of the book gives the reader a simple but sophisticated, science-based set of questions to apply to real-world pathology and therapeutic goals.

Jeffery Smith's work as a psychiatrist, therapist, teacher, and international leader is driven by a mission to improve the field of psychotherapy by combining science with the humanism clients need.

How Psychotherapy Works

Navigating the Therapeutic Space with Confidence

Jeffery Smith

Routledge
Taylor & Francis Group
NEW YORK AND LONDON

Designed cover image: Rod Long, Unsplash

First published 2027
by Routledge
605 Third Avenue, New York, NY 10158

and by Routledge
4 Park Square, Milton Park, Abingdon, Oxon, OX14 4RN

Routledge is an imprint of the Taylor & Francis Group, an informa business

ISBN: 9781041025177 (hbk)
ISBN: 9781041025160 (pbk)
ISBN: 9781003619659 (ebk)

DOI: 10.4324/9781003619659

Typeset in Bembo
by Deanta Global Publishing Services, Chennai, India

Dedication

To helpers with the courage and honesty to keep questioning and growing and to my clients who have bravely shared their experiences and shaped the core of what I have learned about psychotherapy and human nature.

Contents

List of figures *xi*
Acknowledgments *xii*
Author's Note *xvi*
Foreword *xx*

Introduction: How We Got Here and Why the Time for Change Is Now 1

1 A Foundation for Success 10

2 Psychotherapy Treats Entrenched Maladaptive Patterns 20

3 EMPs Come in Layers 39

4 Inner Selves, the Authors of EMPs 52

5 The Plan 67

6 Inside Every EMP 83

7 Five Key Questions: A Method for Seeking Accurate Empathy 100

8 Three Mechanisms of Change 114

9 Bringing Affect into the Room 126

10 The Art of Disconfirmation 137

11 Hope, Motivation, and Development 153

12 Boundaries and Pitfalls 168

13 How This Framework Supports Many Therapies 179

14 The End of a Voyage and the Beginning of a New One 195

Appendix: Biology Meets Psychology—Some Notes *205*
Index *211*

List of figures

2.1	Two Minds	23
2.2	EMPs: From the inner mind to the outward response	30
2.3	Until You Run into Resistance, You're Not Doing Work	35
3.1	Layered Protections	40
4.1	Two Direct Products; Three Indirect Via Consciousness	64
6.1	Outputs of the Basic Inner Mind	89
6.2	Margaret's Bottom Level EMP	94
7.1	Five Key Questions	102
8.1	Three Change Mechanisms	115
13.1	Three Clinical Objectives	183

Acknowledgments

Helen Singer Kaplan gave grand rounds during my residency at Albert Einstein College of Medicine and described giving behavioral homework for sex therapy, then using psychodynamic principles to understand why the couple didn't do the homework. That was my first introduction to psychotherapy integration. I didn't forget, which means I was already attuned to the idea.

Sibylle K. Escalona ran a child development research elective in my residency, observing 18-month-old children and interviewing their mothers. That was the beginning of a lasting interest in psychological development.

Margaret Mahler, R.D. Laing, John Searles, Heinz Kohut, Otto Kernberg, Daniel Stern, and John Bowlby. I studied each of them as I sought to understand development and intrapsychic dynamics, but especially development.

Suzanne K. Langer, a philosopher, wrote about the richness of nonverbal communication. My father was a professor of philosophy, interested in aesthetics, so it was not a surprise that he had her book, *Philosophy in a New Key* on his shelves. Somewhere early in my professional development, I came upon that book and recall a memorable boost to my interest in the language of the nonconscious mind.

Milton Rosenbaum visited the residency in the summer and showed us how to talk to patients. In his demonstration interviews, he would help patients talk about themselves, then, about halfway through the interview, he would put his foot on the rung of the patient's chair, lean in, and start the real core of the interview.

Leon Balter taught Freudian theory with precision and clarity. I loved his class, and it set me on a long journey to think about how to state theory in a way that was no longer restricted to one orientation.

Joel Kovel. Joel was my best supervisor in residency. He told me to "Mix it up with the patient." He was smart, flexible, and tuned in.

Maj-Britt Rosenbaum, Milton's daughter in Law, reached out when I was first starting a practice and freely gave me the biggest boost in my early practice.

Michael Blumenfield persistently pushed me to be active in the American Psychiatric Association. He is a valued mentor and supporter, known for publishing *Shrink Talk*, a blog, and now a book.

Robert Feinstein, who consults now on psychotherapy training, asked me to teach residents how to combine behavioral and psychodynamic techniques in the early 2000s. That led me to SEPI, the Society for the Exploration of Psychotherapy Integration and fueled my interest in what tied all therapies together.

In 2010, I started a blog for clients. I am grateful for a reader's question that turned the blog into a forum for clients who were experiencing intense attachment to their therapist. From there, reader's stories of therapeutic disasters led me to shift my professional mission to helping therapists do better with intense emotions.

In 2015, I changed the direction of my blogging with a new domain, Howtherapyworks.com, aimed at helping therapists.

Bruce Liese, under the SEPI presidency of John Norcross, recruited me to bring back to life the long-dormant SEPI newsletter, "The Integrative Therapist." I endeavored to make it into an informal but exciting forum for ideas.

Irvin Yalom wrote the textbook of group therapy I read as a resident. He is also author of *The Gift of Therapy: An Open Letter to a New Generation of Therapists and Their Patients.* That book was my inspiration in wanting to write a companion for therapists, but one that would be helpful by explaining what was going on underneath.

George Silberschatz, clinical professor at the University of California (UCSF) School of Medicine, is the psychological thinker whose ideas come the closest to my own in understanding how clients develop the problems psychotherapy is designed to treat.

Bessel van der Kolk's talks and book, *The Body Keeps the Score* influenced me to pay attention to the body and how movement generates experiential information that communicates directly with the inner mind.

Bruce Ecker wrote the book that introduced me to memory reconsolidation. I had described the phenomenon in my paper of 2004 but thought the mechanism of transformational change was extinction. That turned out to be incorrect. What I heard at a conference told me in a flash that what I had witnessed was really memory reconsolidation. That night, I devoured his book, *Unlocking the Emotional Brain*. He is still the only one I know of who has recognized the two schemas in a survival circuit and who thinks in terms of the threat processing and the flow of information.

Richard Lane, a researcher and scholar at the University of Arizona is a pioneer in recognizing the importance of memory reconsolidation. After reading his seminal 2015 paper, I walked into a SEPI conference in Dublin, and there he was. He has been a friend and colleague since.

Benjamin Johnson was a doctoral candidate when he volunteered to co-write a paper and patiently helped with a first article, where we presented the framework at the core of this book. It was rejected, but persistence eventually led to a third article, the intellectual basis of this book, being published in the Journal of Psychotherapy Integration (Smith 2025). He also took the fine portrait of me featured in this book.

Les Greenberg started out wanting to develop a theory that would tie multiple therapies together. He ended up pioneering Emotion Focused Therapy, where he did close observation and developed important concepts about emotion. I wanted to further his direction in building the framework of this book.

Marvin Goldfried was a co-founder of SEPI, and one of the first, especially from a behavioral background, to endorse my thinking in the YouTube video organized by Gregg Henriques (see below). I am grateful for his one-word endorsement of this book.

Jack Anchin welcomed me into the group of SEPI members involved in a new approach to psychotherapy integration, the Unification Movement, looking for a metatheoretical umbrella that would incorporate and embrace the best of many therapies.

Gregg Henriques is a former President of SEPI, another member of the Unification Movement and notable clinical philosopher. I am indebted to his strong support. Together we did the remarkable YouTube video with Marvin Goldfried, an early and remarkable milestone in coming to consensus on the common bases of all psychotherapies.

Jeffrey Magnavita and André Marquis, co-authors of Unifying Psychotherapy, have lent me wonderful support. Andre mentored me for the paper that forms the foundation of this book, and Jeffrey featured me in another video, part of a series called "Eminent Psychotherapists Revealed" on YouTube.

Amelie Southwood worked with me tirelessly to record 25 episodes of the "How Therapy Works" podcast, a year-long course in integrated psychotherapy.

Stephen Hayes is one of the behaviorists I most admire for his clinical wisdom and openness to sciences outside our field. He has supported the idea of survival circuits as sources of the problems we treat.

Eric Plakun is the founder of the Psychotherapy Caucus of the American Psychiatric Association. Eric has been a mentor and supporter as I have been elected to the helm of that organization of 1,600 psychiatrists who believe in the importance of psychotherapy in our profession.

Kiki Kennedy, a psychiatrist recognized for her active advocacy within our field, welcomed me into the Psychotherapy Committee of GAP, the Group for the Advancement of Psychiatry, an important think tank for our profession, and charged me with organizing a group to advise the ACGME on requirements for residency training in psychotherapy.

Anne Ruble, former chair of the Psychotherapy Committee of AADPRT, the American Association of Directors of Psychiatry Residency Training, has been a supportive and helpful colleague as we have worked to improve residency training.

Donna Sudak co-authored a seminal paper with Eric Plakun on the "Y" model for psychotherapy training. She has been a knowledgeable supporter and source of wisdom on the psychotherapy training of psychiatrists.

Heather Fryer has been my coach during from the start of this book project, helping me find my direction and priorities.

Anna Moore, Routledge's acquisition editor welcomed me in, having worked with many of the people I most respect on books about the things I care about.

Lisa Shiroff, my multi-talented editor fixed the manuscript according to things like the Chicago Manual that I've heard of, but don't understand.

Sharon Katz brought her artistry and graphic talent to invent and design the book's figures.

And Claude Smith, who has patiently and tirelessly supported my work.

There are so many more who have helped and influenced my career and thinking. Thank you, to all those I have not mentioned by name.

Author's Note

IS THIS BOOK FOR YOU?

All therapists have doubts and all of us want to be better therapists. My aim in writing this book is to combine my broad experience as a therapist and teacher with insights from modern neuroscience to give you the confidence we all need to do our best work. In short, by identifying core principles, I want to make it as easy as possible to know from moment to moment what's going on and what needs to happen next.

This book is a companion for therapists and other professionals at any stage of their careers. It frames the work we do in a way that is firmly grounded in science, while capturing the art and warmth of working with the inner mind and nonverbal meanings that are critical to success. In addition, it is friendly to diverse therapies, bringing them under one big roof, where understanding how they work allows for thoughtful matching of techniques to the individual as well as guidance for further refinement.

What has stood in the way of this kind of simplicity is that the field of psychotherapy remains in what Thomas Kuhn called its "preparadigmatic" phase. That means we have yet to agree upon the basic principles that underlie what we do. As a result, every therapy has had to invent its own constructs and explanations. The resulting divisiveness makes learning overcomplicated, creates anxiety for therapists, and is confusing for clients. Today we can do better. Together, we will build a picture of how psychotherapy works that will come to mind as you sit with clients and that will be there to guide your choices of what to say and do.

The answer to psychotherapy's divisiveness is that it's time to look at the infrastructure that underlies all therapies. As we do so, we will be able to explain where the problems we treat come from as well as how words, nonverbal communication, and relationships are able to bring about lasting change. Our voyage together will lead to an accessible (and teachable) way to visualize what is happening as we work with our clients. This is made possible by bringing together three critical elements:

1. We narrow our subject to only those maladaptive patterns that psychotherapy is designed to treat. This is in contrast to the more common practice of looking at "disorders," which represent unordered and confusing mixtures of biological and psychological symptoms.
2. We focus on the mind/brain as an information processing organ, which is both the source of maladaptive patterns and the primary domain where psychotherapeutic change takes place.
3. We take advantage of recent science from widespread sources including evolutionary biology, learned fear, predictive processing, and how nonverbal information is stored. All this will go into building an easy-to-understand picture of how problems form and how psychotherapy helps clients trade old patterns for healthier ones.

Finally, by becoming familiar with how the nonconscious mind works, we will understand the art of psychotherapy. We will see that empathy and intuition are essential if we are to reach into the nonverbal regions of the mind where schemas, the final targets of psychotherapy, are located. To concretize this, the book will offer Five Key Questions as a guide to gaining "accurate empathy," an ever deepening, emotionally engaged, understanding of the individual that naturally leads to fulfillment of requirements for transformational change.

I hope you will join me on this voyage. My promise is that you will become a better observer and a more confident helper by understanding and appreciating the inner mind where problems develop and where healing and growth take place.

AM I THE ONE TO TELL THIS STORY?

Yes, I have the credentials. Stanford undergrad, UCLA med school, SUNY Upstate internship in internal medicine, Albert Einstein residency in psychiatry, and my current appointment as Clinical Professor of Psychiatry at New York Medical College. Beyond that, I am Leader of the American Psychiatric Association's Psychotherapy Caucus and immediate Past President of SEPI, the Society for the Exploration of Psychotherapy Integration. I am currently on my 136th blog post for therapists and have lectured around the US and abroad. In addition, my recent peer-reviewed article (Smith, 2025) presents the core concepts this book is based on.

But those aren't the real reasons why this book is trustworthy. I'm a career clinician. I never specialized, so I have seen everything. I have been happy to work with whoever came through the door, including the difficult and unusual cases. If I were an academic, I would have had to narrow my view to a specialized niche. Being a general psychiatrist/therapist I have enjoyed full freedom of thought and an openness to new territory. I'm fiercely critical of my own work and ideas, and they must withstand my own and others' scrutiny. The thinking you will find here is born from a longstanding passion for continuously questioning and deepening my understanding of what is going on. At the same time, I keep up with the science and with the work of others. My motto is a quote attributed to Einstein: "Make everything as simple as possible but not simpler."

WHAT TO EXPECT

This book is the one I wished I had when I started my career. The order in which the chapters unfold is intended to maintain your interest while you learn with each page. I try to alternate chapters that have a heavier emphasis on science and theory and those that give more of a feel for how this works in practice. We'll start in the first chapter by discussing an effective mindset. Then we move to building a unified picture of the problems (subunits of pathology) that all psychotherapies are designed to treat. To describe those, I'll introduce the one jargon term: Entrenched Maladaptive Patterns (EMPs), the problem patterns of behavior and experience that psychotherapy is designed to treat. As we develop a composite picture of the vast range of EMPs, we'll understand why we humans have them, where they come from, and how they are created. That will lead us to identifying those parts of the mind that are the authors of these problems and how we can get personal with them.

Next, we'll look at the inner workings of EMPs because that will lead us to what, exactly, needs to change and how change happens. Learning the requirements for transformative change will take us full circle to the many things clinicians already do to make change happen. I say full circle, because the science ultimately explains and supports what brilliant intuition and experience have taught during more than a century of psychotherapy practice.

In Chapter 7, I'll introduce the Five Key Questions, a practical yet sophisticated way to build understanding in sessions. Then we'll dig into knowing how to make transformative change happen. By understanding just what is going on, we'll be able to further improve our use of existing techniques.

In the subsequent chapters, we'll continue to look at helpful skills and important aspects of the conversations we have with clients. In Chapter 11, we'll focus on motivation and how it keeps the process of therapy going. In Chapter 12, we'll discuss how to maintain a safe and positive relationship, and in Chapter 13, we will see in detail how the principles we have learned are embedded in every brand of therapy.

In the final chapter, I present a summary of the contents of the book using each of the Five Key Questions to make sense of example cases. At the end, in the appendix, I share some personal notes on the difficult area where pathologies have a substantial biological basis yet involve psychotherapy to a significant extent. The discussion will also touch on how psychopharmacology enters into the picture.

I hope you enjoy this voyage. I sincerely believe this book will lead you to think differently about psychotherapy for the rest of your career.

REFERENCE

Smith, J. (2025). Psychotherapy integration from the bottom up: A unifying, science-based view of psychotherapy's infrastructure. Journal of Psychotherapy Integration, 35(4), 256–271. https://doi.org/10.1037/int0000371

Foreword

Close to a century and a half ago, Freud began what was referred to as the "talking cure." Since that time, we have learned an enormous amount about how therapy can reduce symptomatology and improve psychological functioning. Unfortunately, there has been a proliferation of different schools of thought of how to best do this, and our siloed approach to intervention unfortunately places more emphasis on who, rather than what, is right. The field of psychotherapy has finally come to the point where it is beginning to reach some consensus, and this most impressive contribution by Jeffery Smith represents an important step in making that happen. In this significant volume, Smith has distilled the essence of the therapeutic change process, bringing the field of psychotherapy to a new level of effectiveness.

Marvin R. Goldfried, PhD
Distinguished Professor of Psychology (ret.)
Stony Brook University
Co-Founder of SEPI, the Society for the Exploration of Psychotherapy Integration

Introduction

How We Got Here and Why the Time for Change Is Now

I sat waiting with a handful of resident psychiatrists. It was my first job, and I had been asked at the last minute to fill in for another attending doctor to lead a teaching exercise. I was to interview a patient and lead the discussion afterward.

The door opened, and a resident entered with a diminutive brunette woman who sat quietly and stared at the floor. I asked her some benign questions to learn a little about her. She was in the hospital after threatening suicide and was unhappy in her marriage but couldn't say much about what the trouble was. Sensing that this line of questioning might be too much for her to handle during a first interview, I moved on and asked about her life. She explained that she worked for the power company and was doing okay in her job. Then I asked about her background. She got up without a word and left the room. One of the residents followed her.

I opened the discussion to talk about what had just happened but was soon interrupted. Suddenly the door reopened, and she returned. I was surprised, but even more so, I was impressed by her pluck and courage. We completed the interview and discussion, and I knew I wanted to be her therapist.

A year later, the opportunity came. It turned out that she had lived a tumultuous early life. Her mother was psychotic and frighteningly abusive. Her father had abandoned the family when she was eight, leaving her and a younger brother to live with her mother. At 16 years, she left her family to enter a Children's Aid Society home for girls. Eventually, she found her job at the power company, married, and had one child.

In our weekly sessions, she was quiet and emotionally flat. Whenever I moved the conversation toward her early experiences of abuse, anger

DOI: 10.4324/9781003619659-1

flared, and she would shut down. The outbursts seemed to come from a different part of her, one that knew more than she wanted to face. I came to believe she was dissociative. One time, with a huge swipe of her arm, she cleared my desk but spared the one object that was breakable. There was someone inside watching out for me.

Four tumultuous years in, I knew she had multiple personalities and that another self was guarding the darkest secrets of her abuse. All this happened before there was professional literature or guidance on treatment for cases like this. We had to learn on our own, along with some help from Freud's early writings when he wrote cogently about trauma therapy. I did my best, and little by little, she became less angry.

The day came when her first trauma memory surfaced. She sat on the floor, seemingly barely aware of her surroundings, and began to recount what had happened. There was nothing for me to say, but I put in a word or sound here and there to remind her that we were still in the present, not back when she was eight. The terror and hurt she expressed seemed as if the experiences were happening right then. I prolonged the session. After two hours, she was exhausted and feeling a dull ache, but the horror and immediacy of her pain were gone. They were gone permanently.

That was my first encounter with transformative change. It was rapid, complete for that part of the trauma, and the healing did not require further reinforcement. That first, terrible trauma was forever behind her. It remained a sad memory, but nothing more than that.

A few years later, Castonguay (2006) wrote about transformative change and the factors that contributed to it, but he was unable to precisely explain how and why it worked. Being intent on understanding the why, I had written a paper (Smith, 2004) describing the same kind of dramatic change and providing a tentative explanation based on extinction, a change mechanism I will describe in detail in Chapter 8. We'll see that I got the mechanism wrong, but that's because the neurochemistry of the actual mechanism, *memory reconsolidation*, had only just been brought to light by Karim Nader (Duvarci & Nader, 2004) and was practically unkown to therapists. Since then, Bruce Ecker (2022), as well as Richard Lane (2020), have been champions of memory reconsolidation as the explanation for transformative change. That work will be central to the framework underlying this book.

With my client, we went on to recover and process additional horrific experiences. They seemed to come up every four years in the therapy. She enrolled in a day hospital during the most difficult times. Eventually, she secured government funding to attend college and later social work school. By the time of her graduation, her therapy had wound down, and she was functioning well in her new career.

I noticed that the drain on her self-esteem, typical of most survivors of early trauma, took much longer to resolve. It was far more resistant to change than the pain of her horrific traumas. This left me puzzled. I was witnessing more than one change process, but nowhere in my training had that possibility been mentioned. A desire to explain what I had noticed remained at the center of my curiosity as my career evolved. We'll learn more about this second change process in Chapter 5, in the section on inner critics and how they tarnish self-esteem.

From that early case and many others, I learned what residency hadn't taught about trauma. I learned about inner selves, about development, about knowing what to do next, and, most recently, about the science that has finally reached the level of explaining transformative change. What you will find here is a fresh and modern approach to integrating clinical observation and recent science into a framework that will guide you as you sit with your clients.

Teaching psychotherapy to residents became a regular part of my professional life. As I continued to pursue my most passionate interests, I never stopped refining how to express what I was learning in ways that could bring clarity to others. Over these past decades, my vision of psychotherapy has evolved from what I was taught in traditional psychodynamic training. Now I view therapy as a broad range of techniques that support a few fundamental processes and are powerfully useful in helping people improve their varied and fascinating lives. How many professions are so privileged that they are never boring? Among them, I'm sure this is the very best.

EPISTEMOLOGY AND EVIDENCE

For those who are interested in the intellectual underpinnings of the book, what follows are some notes about the ground I stand on. This book, while timely and relevant, does not rest on quite the same foundation as its peers. What you will find here is a fresh assembly of concepts from several areas of science within and beyond psychology. These include evolutionary biology, the neuroscience of information, and the neurobiology of change. Putting these ideas together will lead to a fresh and modern framework for understanding what a century of intuition and experience has taught us to do. It will fill in the area where existing theories have, of necessity, been at their weakest, explaining precisely how words, nonverbal communication, and relationship lead to change.

I am not introducing any brand-new principles, so why has this book not already been written? The reason has to do with the history of the science of psychotherapy. As Thomas Kuhn (1962) describes the development of contemporary sciences, each one begins in a preparadigmatic phase, where there is no agreed-upon foundation, and one person's conjecture is as good as another's. Every science started that way. Theories to explain matter, such as earth, air, fire, and water, were elegant constructions of the imagination. People chose which school to join based not on evidence for their theories, but on the persuasiveness of their founders. Eventually, experiments began to show which ideas held up, and which did not. From there, basic paradigms evolved and coalesced. Most disciplines moved to the stage of *normal science*, where the work no longer consists of building the basic framework, but in using experiments to fill in the details.

The science of psychotherapy is in an unusual place. On the level of a widely accepted paradigm, we are not there yet. We have remained stuck with multiple competing theories, none of which have been based on solid science. However, the field has acted as if it has already transitioned to normal science, when it hasn't. *Normal science* means experimentally filling in the details, and that has become the expected norm, in spite of the fact that we still don't have a solid base. The result is a focus on mediators and correlations such as common factors, which meet high standards of proof but don't help us explain what is going on. *Evidence-based* has been taken as the criterion for scientific validity but refers, again, to statistical correlations, while remaining silent about the underlying mechanisms.

The truth is that, as a science, psychotherapy is still in its early stages, where the goal is finding consensus on how and why words, nonverbal communication, and relationship can bring about transformational healing and growth.

The view presented here is appropriate for the early stages of building a paradigm. Like the theory of relativity when first presented, the framework proposed here offers coherent explanations and is consistent with observation but has yet to be fully tested. On the other hand, it offers a new beginning, a foundation compatible with existing therapies and supportive of what we already know, but now underpinned by science bearing on cause and effect. Furthermore, for both clinical and teaching purposes, we can use it to guide and even improve known techniques by understanding how they support underlying change mechanisms.

Beyond offering confirmation of what is already known, clarity about mechanisms of action has multiple benefits. It provides a kind of Rosetta Stone to translate between diverse conceptualizations. Beyond current practice, it clears a path for expanding the therapist's palette of techniques so we can better match treatment to client specifics. Understanding change mechanisms invites us to further refine existing ways to bring about change. And finally, it provides a basis for future research across therapeutic silos, for example, comparing ways of achieving what will be highlighted as three final objectives of psychotherapy: Expanding the client's repertoire of healthy responses, putting the old, maladaptive pattern in an active state, and delivering new, disconfirming information to the subcortical locations where it can lead to transformational change. We'll discuss those three clinical objectives in Chapter 8 and then in Chapter 13, when we look at how the present framework fits with diverse therapies and orientations.

A DIFFERENT LEVEL OF ABSTRACTION

Besides turning to science outside the field of psychology, the phenomena underlying psychotherapy are approached here from an unusual point of view. Like the approach adopted by Ecker (2024), this book seeks commonalities at the level of information processing and signaling. The discussion begins with an understanding of what Ledoux (2021) calls *survival circuits*, systems evolved for the protection of the individual and the species. Compared to the level of traditional theories, where important incompatibilities have prevented integration, this lower level of abstraction brings to light an infrastructure common to all therapies. Examining the mind's threat processing and the flow of information represents a lower level of abstraction that is applicable to existing therapies without contradicting their proprietary constructs. In doing this, we pass underneath the usual areas of incompatibility between opposing orientations of psychotherapy. Conceptualizations like intrapsychic conflict and cognitive restructuring are not addressed directly, but the mechanisms underlying them are examined and connected with what therapists do.

One factor that may have slowed progress in the science of psychotherapy is resistance to studying information processing that occurs outside of consciousness. While the behavioral orientation has remained reluctant to form hypotheses about nonconscious processing, the field of evolutionary biology has been open to active discussion of the advantages of various adaptations, acknowledging that definitive proof is often not possible. Within cognitive psychology, considerable work has been done on System 1 thinking (Kahneman's *thinking fast*), which, by definition, takes place outside of consciousness and is assumed to be purposeful. This acknowledgment of purposefulness is consistent with Joseph Ledoux's (2021) concept of automatic, nonconscious survival circuits architected for species survival and procreation. In the present synthesis, these concepts are brought together to examine how nonconscious processes can be considered responsible for protective functions of the mind, which are the source of the problems psychotherapy is designed to treat. The well-studied neurophysiology of fear processing is used to explain how existing techniques and concepts support fulfillment of the conditions required for known neurophysiological change mechanisms.

Where prominent theoreticians like Steven Hayes (2018) refer to Ledoux's survival circuits in discussing the origins of psychological problems, the present framework goes a bit further to embrace the accumulated wisdom of the psychodynamic orientation's century-plus of indirect study of nonconscious information processing. This is brought to bear in proposing and examining hypotheses about the purposefulness and functions of the nonconscious mind's protective operations.

FROM NONVERBAL MEANING TO WORDS AND BACK

Another epistemological issue that enters the discussion is the concept of *accuracy* and how it applies slightly differently to verbal and nonverbal communications. A picture is, perhaps, the quintessential nonverbal communication. The images of Michelangelo and Van Gogh can be said to be accurate in that the artists' mastery of their medium allows them to communicate precisely how they envisioned a subject and its meaning. We can seek an understanding of those meanings, but only approximately. Empathy, and accurate empathy in particular, appear in this discussion as approximations of our clients' experience. Compared with formal verbal logic, the level of accuracy is woefully inadequate. On the other hand, in terms of the richness and volume of meaning exchanged, accurate empathy goes far beyond what the denotative meanings of words can express. The point is that in the field of psychotherapy, not to mention the fuzzy logic of artificial intelligence (AI), accuracy, and even "truth" may need to be viewed in a different way than what has been assumed as the gold standard, the truth of formal, traditional logic. In psychotherapy, as in art, imagery and metaphor can be thought of as the height of accuracy, if not truth.

Psychotherapy involves both the client's efforts to translate nonverbal meaning into words and our efforts to understand those word pictures and to communicate back in our own verbal and nonverbal terms. We are often working with metaphors as the best available ways of capturing meaning. As long as we are talking about meaning, then the term accuracy is a valid measure of how well our approximations and our clients' approximations manage to meet in the middle. Humans are remarkably able to communicate on that level, and when we do, we instinctively experience a Hellen Keller moment of connection. When those meetings happen, a channel for the communication of *information* is opened up with the inner mind and that is when enduring change takes place.

LIMITATIONS OF THE SCIENCE

The standards of proof in science might be compared to those in the law. In civil cases, the standard is *the preponderance of the evidence.* Criminal cases, however, demand a higher standard: *beyond a reasonable doubt.* In normal science, the standard for experiments should be similar to the criminal standard, beyond a reasonable doubt. That is where we seek "p values" of less than .001. In this book, consistent with the idea that our science is still seeking consensus on a paradigm, the standard should be more like the civil one, the preponderance of the evidence. Where evidence exists, it is cited, both here and in my more formal article (Smith, 2025). In other instances, conceptualizations and working hypotheses are based on observations accessible to any experienced clinician.

In many instances, it is clinically and heuristically valuable to consider a principle to be universal. When a principle is always true, we can use the logic of elimination. Conclusions can be based on ruling out possibilities other than the one we end with. This only works when the possibilities are limited. Thus, even if there is some room for doubt, being able to state a universal principle can narrow the possibilities to a finite list, making it possible to rule out those that don't apply and to home in on the one that is most likely. This is the basis of "differential diagnosis," seeking the most likely among a limited list of possibilities. In our case, universal principles are helpful in evaluating possible formulations or the most likely function of a symptom. An important example in this book is the idea that entrenched maladaptive patterns (EMPs), subunits of pathology, are *always* derived from responses to threats in contrast to opportunities. Making that universal statement greatly simplifies building a working hypothesis about what specific threat an EMP was originally created to mitigate. Similarly, the section below about change mechanisms acknowledges the lack of proof beyond reasonable doubt, but presents an argument based on the logic of elimination for the role of memory reconsolidation in psychotherapy. Overall, despite these limitations, the aim here is to present an understanding of reality that is consistent with multiple sources, including contemporary science, existing psychotherapies, and clinical experience. Once an understanding has passed those tests, it still needs to be useful for navigating the infinite variety of situations encountered in helping clients. Those are the standards by which the ideas presented here should be measured. Proof beyond reasonable doubt may have to wait.

THE ARGUMENT FOR MEMORY RECONSOLIDATION

Perhaps the most central argument of the book is the one that MR plays a fundamental role in psychotherapy. At the same time, the kind of proof one would expect in a normal science has not been demonstrated. Elsey et al. (2018) suggest criteria to prove that MR is the cause of a clinical change in functioning. To date, those criteria remain beyond reach. While the action of memory reconsolidation has been amply proven in animal models and in humans under laboratory conditions, absolute chemical proof of its role in therapeutic change under clinical conditions has not been possible so far. How, then, can it be responsible to assert here that MR has a role in our work?

Bruce Ecker's logic of elimination is relevant. Many clinicians, including myself, have observed transformational change taking place rapidly and remaining solidly in effect without further reinforcement. Ecker argues by elimination that there is no other known mechanism for producing such results. His reasoning is that, given that the action of MR is to rewrite the procedural memory at the heart of problem schemas, and that there is no other known way to explain similar results, then observed transformative change must be due to the action of MR. Therefore, it seems reasonable to accept provisionally the hypothesis that MR is, in fact, responsible for these instances of change.

For further confirmation, we can add that observed clinical circumstances resulting in transformative change closely match the requirements found in the laboratory to lead to confirmed memory reconsolidation. Those requirements are the activation of old procedural memory juxtaposed with exposure to disconfirming information. Clinically when we see those two conditions fulfilled, we are also likely to observe transformational change, sometimes dramatically and sometimes to a lesser extent. The more fully the conditions are met, the more likely a dramatic change. Furthermore, the fulfillment of these same conditions can be seen as embodied in essentially every effective psychotherapy. Even without absolute proof, the observed phenomenon is highly valuable in a clinical context.

Given the immense value of understanding the universal underlying mechanisms by which psychotherapy works and of moving away from the divisiveness and competitiveness of the preparadigmatic phase of our science, it is arguably time to make use of hypotheses presented here while science continues to work on more absolute and detailed testing and evidence.

CONCLUSION

If you have not skipped this discussion, then I hope it has been of interest. Now, however, it's time to leave the philosophy of science and dig right into how psychotherapy works in order to gain further confidence in navigating the therapeutic space. I'm excited to accompany you on your voyage, so let's get started.

REFERENCES

Castonguay, L. G. (2006). In L. G. Castonguay & L. E. Beutler (Eds.), *Principles of therapeutic change that work*. Oxford University Press.

Duvarci, S., & Nader, K. (2004). Characterization of fear memory reconsolidation. *The Journal of Neuroscience, 24*, 9269–9275.

Ecker, B. (2024). A proposal for the unification of psychotherapeutic action understood as memory modification processes. *Journal of Psychotherapy Integration, 31*(2), 291–314.

Ecker, B., & Vaz, A. (2022). Memory reconsolidation and the crisis of mechanism in psychotherapy. *New Ideas in Psychology, 66*, 100950.

Elsey, J., Van Ast, V., & Kindt, M. (2018). Human memory reconsolidation: A guiding framework and critical review of the evidence. *Psychological Bulletin, 144*, 797–848.

Hayes, S., & Hofmann, S. (2018). Survival circuits and therapy: from automaticity to the conscious experience of fear and anxiety. *Current Opinion in Behavioral Sciences, 24*, 21–25.

Kuhn, T. S. (1962). *The structure of scientific revolutions*. University of Chicago Press.

Lane, R. D., & Nadel, L. (2020). *Neuroscience of enduring change: Implications for Psychotherapy*. Oxford University Press.

Ledoux, J. (2021). As soon as there was life, there was danger: The deep history of survival behaviours and the shallower history of consciousness. *Philosophical Transactions of the Royal Society B: Biological Sciences, 377*, 20210292.

Smith, J. (2004). Reexamining psychotherapeutic action through the lens of trauma. The journal of the *American Academy of Psychoanalysis and Dynamic Psychiatry, 32*(4), 613–631.

Smith, J. (2025). Psychotherapy integration from the bottom up: A unifying, science-based view of psychotherapy's infrastructure. *Journal of Psychotherapy Integration, 35*(4), 256–271. https://doi.org/10.1037/int0000371

CHAPTER 1

A Foundation for Success

The year was 1965. I, a college freshman, sat in a packed auditorium listening to Paul Tournier, a Swiss psychiatrist and pastoral counselor. I don't remember the contents of his talk, but what stayed in my memory was the way he answered challenging questions from the students. He would listen to a question, then, with an uncanny ability to understand the concern behind it, he would respond in a way that addressed with tact and warmth what they were really asking. I wanted to be able to do that.

Three more years of college, four of medical school, one of internship, and a year of inpatient psychiatry got me to the starting line. It was a hot day at the beginning of July. I still remember the name of the young woman assigned to me for therapy. She said, "I'm not happy." If she had said she was hearing voices, I might have had an idea of what to do or what to say. It was mid-summer, classes hadn't started, and all the supervisors were on vacation on Cape Cod, which meant I had no one to ask for help. Soon, she realized I was not up to the job and dropped out of treatment. I still feel bad about disappointing her. I was personally crushed. It was what I had worked so many years to get to, and I had failed utterly. The thought of giving up did not enter my mind, though, only the determination to learn and get better at what I had dreamed of doing well.

The aim of this book is to pass on what I wished I had back then when I entered the profession. Besides having someone to talk to, what I really would have valued was to understand how psychotherapy works, so that I could have known not only what to do but why and how it would work. Only since the turn of the twenty-first century has science been available to fill in the last gaps in understanding how psychotherapy brings about change. My purpose here is to support you by providing a

DOI: 10.4324/9781003619659-2

clear and memorable framework for understanding, while giving practical ways to put it to work. However, before moving into how to build confidence, I want to share some principles to make the work of helping others a joy and a privilege.

CURIOSITY IS ALLOWED

Humans are naturally interested in other humans. We people-watch; we are fascinated by the way art gives us a glimpse into another's mind; and we never tire of stories about humans interacting with each other and the world around them. But we are often careful not to pry into people's private lives. Curiosity can feel intrusive, so we hold back. As a therapist, how good is it to have a mandate, a powerful and positive reason for following our curiosity and learning about the intimate details of another person's life and experience? We have that privilege because those details will be among the most valuable elements in helping to improve our clients' lives.

It turns out that our curiosity is like a faithful hound, always there to sniff out what we might have glossed over or what is missing. It's the way our inner mind prompts us with questions about things we might not have noticed. It's what makes us want to know the end of the story. We'll go into greater detail about how our inner mind works in later chapters; for now, we'll focus on its remarkable ability to keep track of what's still missing in the mental picture we are building about our client.

Curiosity is a highly sensitive detector of what's important for us because leaving out information is one of the common ways clients and our inner minds avoid the uncomfortable. What's missing from our client's narrative draws a circle around a hot topic that will turn out to be central to our work. So, following our curiosity is not only pleasurable but essential to deepening our understanding. That's not all. The deeper our knowledge of the other person, the more we get interested and the more we feel empathy. And those two qualities, interest and empathy, are among the most powerful elements in building the trust our clients need as they dare to change.

There is a limit. Curiosity is not entirely open-ended because we are there for a purpose. We have a mandate to be curious because it helps us understand, and that is crucial to making things better. Asking specific questions about things that are truly irrelevant to our purpose will feel invasive. Yes, but there is so much that is entirely relevant. How can we tell the difference? Just ask yourself what your motive is in asking. Is it to shed light on the problem and its solution? Or is it more personal? Maybe a good way to think of it is that our mission is to understand the problem and how to harness the client's strengths to resolve it. With that principle in mind, following the thread ever deeper is entirely professional and relevant, including exploration of the breadth and depth of the client's life to learn about the capabilities and resources that will help with progress.

Consistent with those limits, I often don't know the intimate details of my clients' sex lives. But when it is relevant, I ask. People are often private about the abuse they may have suffered, too. That is not something to leave aside. It's good to ask about trauma at the beginning of therapy. We may get a denial or discover that the topic is too hot for right now, but at least we will have indicated an interest and willingness to hear. Why ask at the beginning? People are more ready to accept questions as routine when they come during an initial evaluation. In modern life, we accept all kinds of indignities simply because a database or procedure demands it, so most of us are willing to accept those demands as part of therapy. On the other hand, if we ask a sensitive question later in therapy, it can feel like it came out of the blue. Imagine after a month of sessions, asking, "Do you have a history of abuse?" Then the client will wonder why you asked, and what your motivation is. "Do I look like someone who has been abused?"

So, following our curiosity has some modest limits but leaves a great deal of room to learn about one individual and, at the same time, about the breadth and depth of human life.

BE MORE INTERESTED IN WHAT YOU DON'T KNOW

Following spontaneous prompts from curiosity, I pay attention to knowing what I don't know. It's far more interesting than what I do know because it is likely to lead to a surprise. Humans are especially attuned to novelty, and surprise is a good example. But following our curiosity isn't quite enough. It's even better to make a mental note. Putting what we don't know into our own words makes it more memorable and primes us to pick up hints later that might lead to answers.

Here is an example: After more than a year of treatment with Ellen, something was not working. She began missing sessions and didn't seem to be making much progress from month to month. I had made a mental note that there was something I had yet to understand. There had to be an explanation for her missed sessions and lack of progress. When I'm at an impasse of any kind, I invoke the number one consultant secret: "The answer is staring you in the face, and it has to do with the relationship." Nine times out of ten (or more), that is where the missing perspective lies. In this case, I asked my intuition what might be going on, and it came back with what I said next: "It feels like you are wanting me to help in some way, but it isn't happening."

My client burst out with, "Help! I ask for it a hundred times a day, under my breath. I say, 'Please, I need help, please!'"

That was a turning point. At last, we could discuss how the center of her emotional life was longing for help, while at the same time, she couldn't trust what was offered and blamed herself for needing it. Of course, she had never said that out loud in session. I had to consult my intuition to find a possible answer, then test it by asking to see if my guess was on the right track.

HAVE A WORKING HYPOTHESIS

What makes my first sessions productive is that I aim to have a working hypothesis or *formulation* by the end of the first meeting. Later in the book, I'll call it your *theory*, referring to the explanation you keep in mind for a given client and problem. It is okay that your theory may not turn out to be correct because there is so much we can't know. So, our investment in being right needs to be very light. In fact, I'm happy when my hypothesis turns out wrong because that means I'm about to learn something new. What the hypothesis does is keep me alert for evidence that supports or refutes it, which makes me a better observer. I'm not just taking in random facts; I'm constantly testing and refining a deepening picture.

Clients know I'm doing this. I often share my questions with them and include them as partners in the discovery. As I listen to their history, I'm putting together a story in my own mind. I might recount the story or parts of it to be sure I have it right. Who doesn't want someone to understand them? And for the few who are uncomfortable with this, I'll go gently.

However, I need to make an important distinction here—I am working toward a hypothesis but not applying a label. Labels are not the same as hypotheses. Labeling puts the person in a category, and no one wants to be categorized. A label is an abstraction, meaning that it takes out the meat and leaves only the bones. Labels remove the emotion and the specific facts that make each person's life unique.

A useful hypothesis is concrete and real. "As a five-year-old, you felt so much pain about your dad's bumbling and incompetence that you wanted to be a shining success to redeem his image in your own mind." That is a complex hypothesis, but it is concrete and emotionally tenable.

It is likely to turn out to be true, but there is always room for a deeper or different version. Where did the hypothesis come from? It will arise from the same hidden place as your curiosity. We can call that place our "inner mind," a rich part of every human that we'll learn a lot more about as we go forward.

When a hypothesis comes to mind, I tend to be indulgent and accept it. That sets me up to listen attentively, ready to catch hints of evidence for or against it. I might ask a question to shed a bit more light. If I share an idea, and it doesn't seem to resonate, that means it is either premature or wrong. At that point, I'll put it aside but remember, just in case it re-emerges later.

Carrying these three principles will stand any therapist in good stead. They will bring satisfaction and interest to your sessions as your understanding continues to grow. The next two sections encapsulate how understanding and caring go together, and how they are central to transforming what seems like an interesting conversation into an effective tool for helping turn lives around.

FOLLOW THE COMMON FACTORS

Research shows that relationship factors are strongly associated with therapeutic success (Wampold, 2015). We know intuitively that relationship is important, and now there are strong statistics to confirm it. What's missing is that a good relationship alone is still not enough to untangle each client's web of unique maladaptive patterns. Correlation is not causation. To best use the relationship as an instrument for change, we need to know *why* those correlations exist. What does the relationship do to further the work of psychotherapy? First, let's look at the research, then we'll tackle the why of it. As a preview, we'll soon see that trust is at the center of the common factors and why they are important.

Common factors correlations have, in some ways, been the current high-water mark of the psychotherapy integration movement. In spite of their lack of explanatory power, many programs have settled on common factors as a basis for training. The following relationship elements have been found through multiple studies to contribute to success. Here are the components, listed in approximate order from highest to lowest.

- Expectations and hope (about 15 percent contribution to outcome)
- Consensus on goals
- Therapist empathy
- Quality of the therapeutic alliance

- Positive regard
- Genuineness (lowest at about 5 percent contribution)

Even with this breakdown of the individual aspects of the relationship, these correlations still don't tell us what each one does. The research doesn't help us use them specifically and precisely to fulfill the goal of this book, using a defined and clear-cut understanding to maximize the benefits of what we do. Such explanations need a foundation in theory. In this book, we take advantage of advances in science to propose a hypothesis that explains the underlying infrastructure common to all psychotherapies, one that includes why the common factors help and explains how psychotherapy works to help individuals change their problematic responses to life situations. Let's begin here to make use of theory to look at just what these common factors do.

Why Common Factors Help

The model presented here emphasizes that the inner mind tends to resist change. A consequence is that one of the hardest things clients need to do to move their therapy forward is to take real emotional risks as they work to change beliefs, behavior, and values. Standing up to a controlling partner is an example. It felt like a life-and-death risk to Nancy, a woman who grew up anxious about being loved and accepted by her authoritarian father. The oversized feeling of risk, as we will learn, came from Nancy's inner self, stuck at a time from her past when the angry look in her father's eyes felt far too dangerous, and a confrontation was out of the question.

Because the stakes were so high back then, the sense of danger has remained frozen and has not evolved. At 55 years, it felt just as dangerous to confront her husband or the boss whose eyes had that same narrow look of anger. What would it take for her to express disagreement? Her deep, but outdated fear would require strong support to overcome. It would require more than intellectual clarity, though that helped. It helped, too, that she realized that she had come to a point where she had little to lose in either case. If she allowed her husband to dominate, the marriage was not worth keeping. Similarly, allowing the boss to rule her through fear made the work untenable. The factor that was still missing was one we are all familiar with: the need to feel supported by a connection with another human. The therapeutic relationship brought both intellectual clarity and moral support, enough for her to take a deep breath and go forward.

Realistically, such a change in behavior is not a risk but a test. In the marriage, it was a way to learn whether the partner would tolerate give-and-take in a 50-50 relationship. Will he tolerate a newly evolved relationship with his wife having equal power and voice? How do we help a frightened inner self, tasked with ensuring safety, to allow such a risk? The most important factor is not helping the client calculate the odds. Rather, it is the presence of a trusted other, whose verbal and nonverbal communications validate confidence in her decision.

When we think of the inner self in this situation, we might think of a child going to school for the first time. Children, like clients' inner selves, have no way to imagine or visualize the new experience. They have no way to estimate their chances. Their intellect can offer some help, but they are more familiar with relying on the feeling of support from grown-ups they trust. When we look at the component common factors, the theme running through them is trust. One of the main functions of the common factors is to support trust in the therapist and the process. Here is how common factors promote that kind of trust. The words relating to each common factor are in **bold**.

Expectations and hope: Following a treatment strategy supports positive expectations and hope, especially as steps and milestones are achieved. **Consensus on goals** is a natural result of working together as we listen and seek to understand the client's needs and desires. As we put ourselves in the client's shoes, **therapist empathy** is a natural and expected outcome. Clients appreciate our active interest and become invested in working together, leading to progressive strength in the **therapeutic alliance**. Empathy naturally leads to **positive regard** for the client as we come to appreciate their strengths and accept their less attractive qualities. And finally, the seeking of accurate empathy naturally brings out **genuineness** and discourages artificiality.

All together, these factors support building enough trust in the therapist and the process to take scary emotional risks. Without new experiences to show that the danger is no longer so great, the old fears can't be transformed. With the relationship, we make use of very old, yet healthy patterns learned in early childhood, of relying on trusted others to cope with fears at a time when the child doesn't have the ability to assess the true level of danger.

SEEK ACCURATE EMPATHY

Seeking accurate empathy is a phrase that captures the essence of what makes therapy successful. What's more, it is perhaps the most comprehensive way to express the therapist's job. We are there to seek an ever-deepening accurate empathy. But what is accurate empathy?

The term was coined by Carl Rogers (Clark, 2004) to mean empathy based on a deep, emotionally engaged, and detailed understanding of feelings. That includes not only the feeling, but what triggered it and why. One of my clients prefers the term *complex caring*. It means the same thing but has a less technical spin. Accurate empathy is not an end in itself, but a process of deepening attunement and understanding. And accurate empathy arises when feelings are in the room. As the client is experiencing emotion, we have a sense of knowing them as a unique individual. In pursuing this level of understanding, we also tap into a profound human capacity for connection and bonding.

Accurate empathy is like a Swiss army knife of psychotherapy. It does many things, and all of them contribute to success. The more humans understand one another, the more they care. Understanding helps us bond with and value our clients. For the client, feeling understood promotes a positive relationship. Recognizing client strengths gives the client a stronger feeling of owning those strengths and makes them more available. The trust we earn encourages hope, motivation, and readiness to try out new ways of seeing and reacting. There's more. We'll also see how accurate empathy reaches deep into the mind/brain to activate the processes that bring about enduring, transformational change. As we go forward, we'll see how understanding in detail fulfills requirements for achieving change in the specific problem patterns that are the primary targets of all psychotherapies.

As with the goal of having a working hypothesis, accurate empathy is aspirational. It should be a constantly growing understanding, not one that we should consider achieved and done. We must always be open to different or additional nuances and details at any point in therapy.

As mentioned above, the opposite of accurate empathy is labeling. When we are satisfied with simply naming a feeling or response, we have only applied a label, which makes that aspect of our client's life a commodity, one of many. For good reason, no one likes being put in a category. All humans may face similar challenges in life, but each person's experience is unique. The meanings we make are never quite the same as those of a relative or even sibling. Of course, no person can fully understand another, but part of our inborn equipment is the ability to come remarkably close to understanding the emotions and experiences of other humans.

Accurate Empathy Also Supports Specific Change

Intuitively, it is not hard to understand how common factors related to trust help maintain clients' motivation and willingness to persist in therapy when the work is hard or uncomfortable. What recent science explains is how accurate empathy supports change in each client's unique maladaptive patterns. Going forward, we will learn much more about how this is most likely done via one extensively researched change mechanism, *memory reconsolidation,* allowing rewriting of outdated information stored in memory.

I call memory reconsolidation the *Queen of Change Mechanisms* because it is the only change mechanism known to allow modification of the mental programming that underlies clients' maladaptive patterns (Ecker, 2022). We will learn that memory reconsolidation has two main requirements, each supported by accurate empathy. The first is activation of the old pattern. Seeking to understand often brings up hot topics accompanied by *affect*. When that happens, it means the old pattern has been neurologically activated deep in the inner mind, the subcortical (limbic) brain, where the activation fulfills that first requirement. At the same time, seeking to understand the inner mind's nonverbal thinking brings core beliefs into consciousness, where client and therapist have a chance to see the situation in a bigger perspective. That new perspective, often described as mindfulness, fulfills the second requirement of memory reconsolidation, delivering new, updated meaning that contrasts with the old. In doing so, it sets the stage for rewriting the old programming according to the new information.

The presence of affect has an even more important meaning. It is not only an indication of subcortical activation of the old pattern. Affect also tells us we have succeeded in establishing a two-way communication channel with the inner limbic mind. We receive information about what's going on below the cortex and gain a pathway for sending new information down to those nonverbal, subcortical regions where procedural memory needs to change. Without such a communication channel, the kind of transformative change that is psychotherapy at its best would not be possible.

And, by the way, there is one other common factor that is not about the therapeutic alliance. In-session emotion is also a common factor, found through extensive research to correlate with therapeutic success (Frank, 1971; Whelton, 2004). From the above explanation, we can now begin to understand why this is true. Affect is the therapist's best and most immediate marker to show that relevant activity is going on outside of consciousness, in the subcortical structures most central to the problem patterns being worked with.

With these four principles and our ordinary social skills, we are ready to seek accurate empathy with another human being. The purpose of the remaining chapters is to help you gain a living picture of what your words, nonverbal communications, and relationship are doing and how to put them to work to chart your course with your clients, to help them trade old, outdated patterns for more satisfactory ones.

Key Points

- Use your curiosity to point to what is important that you don't yet know.
- Articulate to yourself what you don't yet know so you will notice it later.
- Keep building a working hypothesis that explains what you see. It will help you learn more and be a better observer.
- Pay attention to the ups and downs of your client's level of trust and motivation.
- Always seek to deepen accurate empathy to help the relationship, and because it lays the groundwork for transformational change.

REFERENCES

Clark, A. (2004). Empathy: Implications of three ways of knowing in counseling. *The Journal of Humanistic Counseling, Education and Development*, *43*, 141–151.

Ecker, B., & Vaz, A. (2022). Memory reconsolidation and the crisis of mechanism in psychotherapy. *New Ideas in Psychology*, *66*, 100945.

Frank, J. D. (1971). Therapeutic factors in psychotherapy. *American Journal of Psychotherapy*, *25*(2), 350–361.

Wampold, B. (2015). How important are the common factors in psychotherapy? An update. *World Psychiatry*, *14*, 270–277.

Whelton, W. (2004). Emotional processes in psychotherapy: evidence across therapeutic modalities. *Clinical Psychology & Psychotherapy*, *11*, 58–71.

CHAPTER 2

Psychotherapy Treats Entrenched Maladaptive Patterns

One might imagine there is agreement about what psychotherapy treats, but no, there isn't. A major consequence of the fact that the field of psychotherapy has yet to adopt a universal scientific basis is that each therapy has had to invent its own idea of what it treats. Obviously, this has created a major hurdle for psychotherapy integration. In this book, we'll consider a solution, identifying entrenched maladaptive patterns (EMPs) as the problems psychotherapy is designed to treat.

We could start with the more familiar concept of DSM (Diagnostic and Statistical Manual of the American Psychiatric Association) disorders, but they are made up of mixtures of problems of biological origin and of the mind. Psychotherapy is designed to deal with the mind, so we will do better to look at *subunits of pathology*, specific ways the mind limits satisfaction in life. But there is a problem. Every therapy still has a different idea of what those subunits are. Here is a list of a few of the things different psychotherapies promise to help change:

- Faulty core beliefs.
- Internal conflicts.
- Unprocessed emotion.
- Problematic schemas.
- Errors in cognition.
- Distorted values.
- Unhealthy responses to trauma.
- Distorted internal models.

Instead of tackling the impossible job of identifying what these various concepts have in common, we are taking a deeper dive to reach a different plane or level of abstraction. We'll reach a level where all therapies do

DOI: 10.4324/9781003619659-3

the same few things to create change. By understanding the *infrastructure* that underlies every therapy, we'll be able to simplify both learning and practice.

As explained in the introduction, this level was not available to the founders of major therapy orientations, which created a relative vacuum. Existing theories are generally not very specific in explaining exactly what words, nonverbal information, and relationships do to bring about change. The missing explanations create an opportunity. At last, using science from this century, we can begin to fill in what was formerly unknowable.

We will be building a picture of psychotherapy as a comprehensive treatment that encompasses a broad range of techniques and concepts. That will allow us the advantage of choosing the best elements for a specific client and situation. The difference is that as we navigate, we will know why those elements are needed and what we want them to do.

The first hint that such a universal infrastructure exists is noticing that all therapies use the same three basic tools: *words, nonverbal communication, and relationship*. With such a limited repertoire, it seems likely that we are aiming for a small group of fundamental change processes. That will turn out to be the case. And just to add one more hint, this is why the effectiveness of all therapies is about the same.

The main thing that makes the approach in this book different from others is that we will focus on the flow of information. Sharing that somewhat unusual vantage point with Bruce Ecker (2024), as we focus on the information processing function of the brain and mind, we will be able to see a group of common features that will greatly help us understand and navigate within the therapeutic space.

Regarding *information* as a basic focus, we could discuss words, but what we communicate is much more than words. It includes tone of voice, connotation, context, body language, and even the furnishings in the room. They are all important in that they convey meaning. *Relationship* is a tool as well. We have already seen in the previous chapter the central role of the therapeutic relationship in supporting the courage to look at oneself honestly and make changes. All three make up the informational content of accurate empathy. From here on in this book, we will consider words, nonverbal information, and relationship as the basic kinds of information that convey meaning in our interaction with clients.

Since *mind* is what we want to work on, and since that word has different meanings, let's choose a definition that suits our purposes. Following Wiggins (2020), we'll think of mind as *the information processing function of the brain*.

The brain and its information processing, shaped over millions of years by evolution, takes in vast streams of data from within and from the outside environment. Both streams are joined and processed to identify *opportunities* and *threats*. When the circumstances are assessed as requiring a response, the mind calculates which response to launch, based on an architecture and organization evolved to improve the odds of species survival and procreation. In other words, the mind processes information to produce *adaptations*. Some are more satisfactory than others.

Let's talk about two minds. The human mind can be thought of as having two parts: an inner, mostly nonconscious part, and the more familiar conscious self. It is especially the nonverbal, automatic, inner mind that psychotherapy aims to change. That's because the inner mind is the first author of the problems psychotherapy treats.

The inner mind produces problems in two ways. First, it controls automatic bodily responses, such as tears and heart rate. Second, it projects thoughts, feelings, and impulses into consciousness, where they have a powerful influence on our "free" choices. The inner mind is tasked especially with survival. Anyone who has tried to lose weight, beat an addiction, or adopt a healthier lifestyle will have experienced the power of those inner thoughts, feelings, and impulses to "protect" us by defeating our efforts at improving our health. Why are they so effective in causing us to override our own positive resolutions? It's because evolution has honed their survival function and with it the ability to steer our voluntary behavior.

FLIPPING OUR VIEW OF THE MIND

Since the Age of Enlightenment, thoughtful people have puzzled over why humans are so often irrational. All this time, we have been getting it wrong. We are basically, fundamentally *irrational*. Our brains are wired for emotion to guide us to safety, based on quick pattern recognition. Rationality is an afterthought of evolution.

The problem is that we think of our personal self as the conscious part because that's what we live with every day, but that is not an accurate picture. A truer version has been around a long time. William James identified two types of thinking including the associative form native to the subcortical inner mind. Before Kahneman's "thinking fast," Seymour Epstein (1994) wrote extensively about the "experiential" mind that is associative, adaptive, and shared with other mammals. A contemporary perspective on this issue, presented by Wiggins (2020), is to flip our

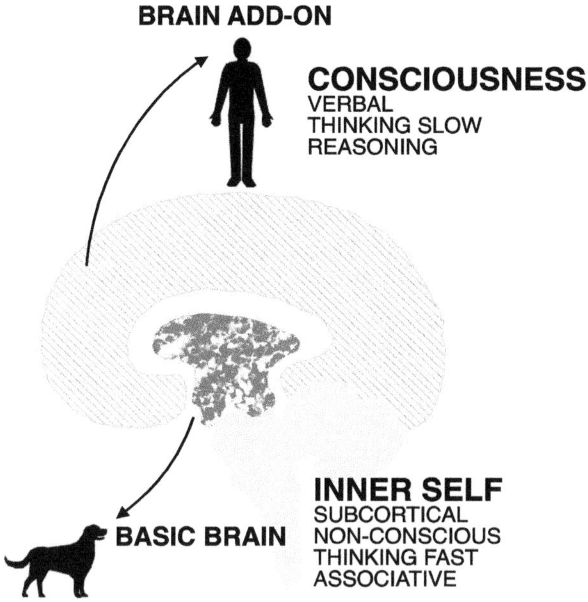

Figure 2.1 Two Minds

point of view to see the human brain from an evolutionary vantage point. That way, the original, basic mind is the nonconscious one and consciousness is an afterthought, an add-on. The basic, nonconscious mind is the one that is anatomically and functionally closest to our mammalian ancestors. It's the one that existed before language and consciousness became available. What is the function of that inner part of the mind? The answer is simple: adaptation to widely varying conditions for the preservation of the species. As in the rest of biology, adaptations are almost always purposeful. Exceptionally, there are features retained from another era that no longer contribute to natural selection or that represent side effects of a healthy adaptation; however, they all make sense in the light of evolutionary advantage and the goal of survival.

With the evolution of primates into humans, the fight for species survival changed drastically and fundamentally. The greatest challenges to other mammals are to avoid being killed by a predator or defeated in a physical battle against a rival. For humans, these concerns have been superseded by the need for social cohesion. We no longer depend on physical strength and big teeth. Instead, we band together to defeat the most powerful predators and fight with other social groups. To help the brain adapt better to these complexities, the cortex became larger, and consciousness was added to our capabilities to permit more subtle responses to the conflicting demands of social life.

As emphasized by pioneer neurophysiologist, Jaak Panksepp (Panksepp & Biven, 2012), the architecture and functioning of various components of the basic inner mind are closely analogous to those of other mammals. As is usually the case in evolution, the old, survival-oriented brain was not abandoned; the basic brain was retained without much physical change but slightly modified to address social safety. For example, physical pain was expanded to include social pain as a potential danger. Other functions, like the worry of isolation or becoming separated, already existed as a way to protect the young mammals from getting lost. They have been adapted to protecting our sense of connection and belonging. Similarly, there already existed systems of motivation and follow-through to make sure goals were achieved. As we will see, these systems work by generating a warning signal, which then triggers the launching of a response. This is still our basic, universal information processing equipment.

In the case of humans, with our incredibly complex social relationships, these same systems continue to operate but have more trouble getting their responses right. An example is the most common phobia, public speaking. If we picture a prehistoric tribe, it might be dangerous to stand on a rock and pronounce some new idea. One could be thrown out of the tribe, and that would mean certain death. On the other hand, in the modern business world, standing up to give a public speech may be essential for economic survival. The long-outdated fear of public speaking could be career-ending. Another common issue involves the potential conflict between the competitive relationship of rivals or enemies and the mutual support of brotherly love, in which siblings or members of the tribe support one another. Both have survival value, but the mammalian survival-oriented inner mind doesn't always know which to favor. For such subtle decisions, evolution demanded even greater computing power.

Overall, the nonconscious, basic mind has the advantage of speed and does an amazing job of coming up rapidly with answers. It also gives us quite reliable physical protection. On the other hand, faced with the incredible complexity of the hyper-social networks that humans depend on, as well as our slow maturation, it is understandable that the basic part of the human mind doesn't always come up with the ideal adaptation.

Conscious Information Processing

Perhaps as a remedy for these deficiencies, humans have evolved what can be thought of as a fancy add-on, the conscious mind. This marvelous invention of nature gives us a new capability, that of being able to *edit* the responses that arise from the basic nonconscious mind. Thus, we are *basically* irrational but have developed *some* ability to reason with our inner mind, which nonetheless remains the source of our strongest emotions, motivation, and instincts for survival. As it often does, nature has created a competition between opposing systems as a way of finding balance between conflicting needs. Having two minds that don't always agree, each with a different point of view, is likely to give our species a better chance of thriving than either mind alone.

What this adds up to is that the irrationality of the human mind and the problems it causes *originate* in the basic, inner mind, and are designed to *influence* the conscious rational mind on the way to being implemented as behavior. This strong influence creates a balance where consciousness and reason have *some* ability to edit and modify the raw responses of the basic, inner mind.

Starting with a modern understanding of the mind and its adaptations, the job of psychotherapy can now be stated as *helping clients trade their mind's less-than-optimal adaptations for more satisfactory ones*. Let's focus, then, on those adaptations and how they can be problematic from the beginning or become so as conditions change.

A Word About Words

Before we move on to our detailed examination of problematic adaptations, we need to be clear about a few terms. I'm going to adopt the informal term, *inner mind* for the basic, nonconscious information processing function that takes place anatomically in the subcortical (under the cortex) parts of the brain. It is true that the inner mind often collaborates with the cortex, but the main decision-making we are concerned with generally happens in subcortical structures like the amygdala and the anterior cingulate. I'm not going to worry much about the details of the anatomy because they are extremely complex and not very well known. More importantly, they don't significantly contribute to our understanding of the *flow of information*, which is the main subject of the discussion. Freud called the same part of the human mind the "unconscious," and later, the "id." I take these as synonyms for what I'll refer to as the "inner mind."

There are also modern studies on the functioning of the inner mind that focus on how it thinks. The most familiar is Kahneman's work on thinking fast and thinking slow—cognitive scientists call these System 1 and System 2, respectively—where thinking fast is associated with the inner mind.

I also like the word *instinctive*. It usually excludes actions that are voluntary, but one of the main points of this book is that many, seemingly voluntary choices are made under the powerful influences of the instinctive mind. And just to add one more twist, the word *implicit* is sometimes used to describe information processing that occurs outside of consciousness. If I use terms other than *inner mind*, I'll specify how they relate to the inner mind as the basic information processing equipment that we, and all other mammals, possess.

OUTDATED ADAPTATIONS

Here are a few examples of maladaptive patterns, chosen to show the enormous variety and quantity of problems within the scope of psychotherapy. Each one represents a strategy adopted by the inner mind in response to a warning signal that predicts potential trouble.

- Avoiding difficult but important interpersonal interactions.
- Recreating unhealthy relationships from the past.
- Self-defeating patterns of behavior.
- Hating or undervaluing oneself.
- Inappropriate shame or guilt.
- Compulsive self-harming behaviors.
- Compulsively using harmful substances.
- Being stuck with anger or sadness that won't resolve.
- Inappropriate anxiety.
- Harming or manipulating others without consent.
- Hopelessness and depression beyond any real basis.
- Resistance to healthy change.
- Chronic pain and muscle tension in the absence of physical pathology.
- Loss of recall of events.
- Multiple identities.
- Inappropriate hypervigilance.

Before we consider their nature, I want to pause and acknowledge the massive contribution these adaptations make to the world's suffering. And, since there is no magic medicine as yet, psychotherapy has a big job to do.

Good and Bad Adaptations

Each of the above maladaptive patterns and others we might encounter in our work can be thought of as products of the inner mind's calculations. The inner mind is doing its very best to protect the client, and if psychotherapy is going to help bring about improvement, there must be at least one potentially better adaptation available.

That doesn't mean the original adaptation was bad from the beginning. In fact, many adaptations start out as very helpful and even necessary. For example, a pattern of mistrust of others might have helped a child deal with a dangerous and manipulative family. Later, the same adaptation, a generally mistrusting attitude, will no longer be ideal. Others, like adapting for survival on a battlefield, may be lifesaving in wartime, but unhelpful in civilian life. Some adaptations like anxiety, obsessive-compulsive disorder (OCD), and depression, have biological roots going back before humans existed and can be over-represented in some individuals. Psychotherapy is not designed to change those, but it can help with adaptations to our own biology. Maladaptive just means that a previously developed solution is less satisfactory than some other available means of coping.

A good way to capture what makes some response patterns targets for therapy is that they are *outdated.* They are no longer the best available adaptation. The aim of psychotherapy, then, can be further refined as *helping clients trade their mind's less-than-optimal adaptations for more satisfactory ones by updating the inner mind's information processing to generate a different and more satisfactory response to the same or similar inputs.*

Do you notice that I'm saying the goal of therapy is to install "more satisfactory" ways of coping? This vague wording gets us out of the position of being arbiters of what is normal. By leaving it up to the client to determine what is more satisfactory, we voice our respect for the client's wishes while recognizing that ultimately it is not our role to decide what is healthy and what is not. We may have our own opinions and can participate in discussions about what the client would prefer, but values are not ours to dictate. This is important for the alliance, as mentioned in the discussion of common factors, since one of them is finding agreement on the goals of treatment.

ENTRENCHED MALADAPTIVE PATTERNS

As noted at the beginning of this chapter, each therapy or orientation proposes its own version of what it treats, but they suffer from the problem of incompatibility with one another. Furthermore, new therapies are primarily developed to address a single type of problem and then expanded to cover other areas. In general, even with expansion, specific therapies still tend not to cover the full range of what can be treated through words, nonverbal information, and relationship.

So far, we have identified the problems that therapy aims to change as adaptations: patterns of response generated by the inner mind that cause pain or loss of functioning either directly or by influencing conscious decision-making. Now we can make use of that universal understanding and give them a name: Entrenched Maladaptive Patterns . Note that these are not the same as the standard DSM disorders. Those disorders are collections of symptoms that tend to cluster together, some more biological and some arising from the mind. For the level of precision that we hope to attain, they are not specific enough. For our purposes, we will need to narrow our focus instead to *subunits of pathology* produced by the inner mind, that is, EMPs. Any one client can exhibit several of them, and we'll discuss in Chapter 3 how they are generally organized in layers.

The EMP concept requires a bit of explanation. *Maladaptive* means these are adaptations that can potentially be replaced with more satisfactory ones. *Pattern* means that they are identifiable products of mind and that they may be repeated. And *entrenched* means that change is not trivial. If they were easy to change, there would be no need for professional psychotherapy. Self-help would be good enough. We'll see later that resistance to change, whether long standing or in the moment, is an important and fundamental property of EMPs. While entrenchment can vary in degree, its power is due to the role of EMPs in assuring the survival of the individual and the species. Instinctively, the inner mind resists letting go of anything designed to promote survival.

To be clear, the term EMP includes both the mind's information processing and the embodiment of its calculations. The inner mind determines what response will be implemented, but the EMP also comprises its outward expression, including automatic bodily manifestations such as changes in breathing and affects like tears, along with thoughts, feelings, and impulses projected into consciousness and the problem behaviors they lead to. Together, the outer manifestations are what we notice and recognize as belonging to a pattern.

Where did the term EMP come from? In earlier teaching and writing, I used the word *dysfunctional*, as in "Entrenched Dysfunctional Patterns." A small group of us from SEPI, the Society for the Exploration of Psychotherapy Integration, including Gregg Henriques and Andre Marquis, agreed that it would be better to call them *maladaptive* in recognition that the basic function of the mind is adaptation. Richard Lane (2020), also a SEPI member, has used the term *recurrent maladaptive patterns* covering much of the same territory but tied more to the psychodynamic orientation. I prefer to avoid jargon terms and acronyms, but we truly need this one to shed light on how, in spite of vast diversity, EMPs have a great deal in common. This is of major importance because their common features are what allow us to build a framework to explain how psychotherapy works to change them, an explanation that both supports and connects diverse therapies by clarifying their common infrastructure.

From What do EMPs Aim to Protect Us?

The simple answer is that EMPs aim to protect us from anything the mind identifies as a threat. The inner, subcortical mind is always scanning for opportunities and threats. Opportunities are not as immediately critical to survival, so patterns aiming to take advantage of them tend to be held less rigidly. For practical purposes, we can eliminate them as triggers for EMPs. Because of that, the problems of concern for psychotherapy can be seen essentially as responses to *threats*. Problems like addiction may have started as pleasure seeking, but by the time they become maladaptive, they are driven not by pleasure but by the need to escape from pain. We don't need to absolutely close the door on opportunities as drivers of maladaptive coping, but we can safely concentrate on threats.

INFORMATION PROCESSING

In protecting us from threats, what all EMPs have in common is the basic inner mind's processing of information. All EMPs begin with a scanning of the environment in the light of the past to identify and predict potential threats. Ledoux (2021) calls these information processing units of the inner mind *survival circuits*. They all have neurological mechanisms to signal a warning that a threat has been spotted, and they all have ways to select a response, launch its implementation, and follow through to be sure it is put into action. This all takes place outside of consciousness through neural firing.

The schemas that determine what is identified as a threat and what response to select are held in a form of memory known as procedural memory, the kind that tells us how to drink from a glass, in contrast to memories of specific experiences. I have already mentioned *memory*

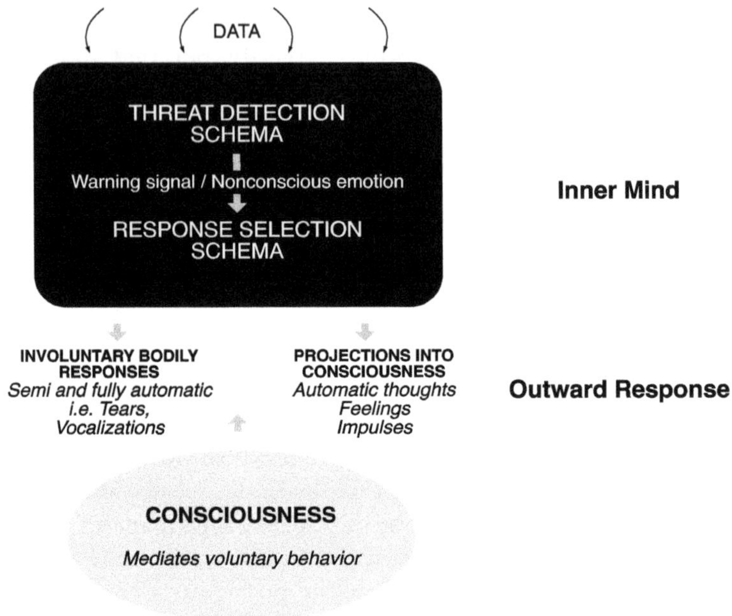

Figure 2.2 EMPs: From the inner mind to the outward response

reconsolidation as a change mechanism. That is the one that can bring about transformational and lasting change to the schemas responsible for predicting threats and selecting responses. The ultimate goal for much of what we do in psychotherapy is to rewrite those schemas, such that the same circumstances lead to a different and improved response.

The Complexity of Human Coping

Before going further, I want to acknowledge the messiness of biology. Philosophers have attempted to create neat generalizations about psychology, for example, by trying to identify the main drivers of behavior. However, it is more typical of biology to be complex and messy, having been shaped over eons by the need to cope with numerous and diverse threats. Other than survival and procreation, the mind/brain can't be reduced to a neat definition of what drives it or why. Similarly, its anatomy and functioning are complex and messy. As Jaak Panksepp (Panksepp & Biven, 2012) describes it, the brain uses different subcortical structures and different neurotransmitters to deal with various kinds of threats. Among them, pain is different from fear, hunger, or panic.

All four lead to energetic responses, but as Panksepp describes, they are embodied in different subcortical structures and use different neurotransmitters. Shame is yet another powerful generator of responses; however, unlike the others, it originates in the cortex. While the study of this anatomical complexity is of great interest to science, for now, it is not very helpful to us. Instead, we will take advantage of the insights that can be generalized about information processing across the full range of EMPs, regardless of which structures and neurotransmitters are involved.

Both Steven Hayes, a behaviorist and originator of acceptance and commitment therapy (2018), and Joseph Ledoux (2021), a pioneering neuroscientist, identify the brain's "survival circuits" as sources of problem patterns. These are the functional units that contain the schemas we want to change. The fact that different ones are located in different parts of the brain is not as important to us as understanding how to rewrite the procedural memory that their neurons are holding.

From these common features, we now turn to some of the ways EMPs are designed as solutions to serious problems in life. Here, the variety is, again, infinite, but we can pick out a few common and important strategies.

THE BREADTH OF STRATEGIES EMPLOYED IN EMPS

At the beginning of the chapter, I provided a list showing the wide variety of problems that psychotherapy is designed to change. Each solution embodies a strategy, and the inner mind is very clever at devising creative ones. I'll put this in perspective with an analogy: in debate classes, students are taught that even if the position they are asked to defend has no good defense, they should still come up with an argument. Especially in childhood, when the inner mind is up against a real problem with no good solution, it will not give up but will find some form of strategy. If necessary, the strategy may be to alter perception rather than reality, but that may be the best that can be done at the time. Let's look at some examples.

One group of threats represents unmet needs. The human brain, especially during formative years, keeps track of what it needs in order to thrive and become its best self. Emotional needs are, for good evolutionary reasons, treated as matters of life and death. These can include the needs for love, to be seen as a unique individual, to receive attention, and for support in dealing with life. Another important time of heightened need comes at the transition from adolescence to adulthood when we take on personal responsibility for our own lives and those of others, all in the face of new and challenging circumstances. You will see an example below with John, whose dreaded neediness threatens to come to the surface because he received a promotion and learned he is going to become a father.

Unmet needs produce entrenched maladaptive patterns when there is no viable way to meet them. If complaining or demanding works to get the need met, then the problem is solved, and no EMP will be created. In contrast, EMPs arise when there is no apparent way to meet the need. The strategies the inner mind adopts may not be very effective, but they are the best it can come up with. One strategy for unmet needs is to seek a substitute, such as food or even self-stimulation, instead of love. In the case of early attachment problems, another solution is to become hyper-self-sufficient so as not to have emotional needs for others at all. Clinically, what we see is *avoidant attachment*. The opposite response to unreliable attachment is clinginess, always seeking reassurance of a connection. That is *anxious attachment*. Another strategy is to wait. Needs can be held in limbo for decades, waiting for someone to fulfill them (and that someone might be you, the therapist). Plans for fulfillment can be put off to the future indefinitely. They surface when the inner mind detects that conditions are, at last, ripe for the need to be met. The inner mind can even tell when the window of possibility is narrowing. You can begin to see the variety and creativity that characterize the inner mind's solutions to serious problems with no immediate solution.

Some threats can best be described as dreaded events or circumstances. They include painful experiences such as bodily harm, separation, defeat, and shame. Once again, EMPs are created when the available protections are not fully effective. They can involve fight, flight, and freeze, which may be more helpful for other mammals faced with predators. In human life, the threats are more often social ones calling for complex patterns of interaction. In these, fight, flight, and freeze may be too simple and less helpful than more sophisticated ways of interacting. Children often learn complex but maladaptive interaction patterns that may have been effective in a dysfunctional family but are not optimal in adult life. "Fawning" is a common example, trying to placate the other.

Strategies can have multiple functions, but many include turning passive into active. Internalizing (identifying with) the attitudes of a bully or perpetrator is a way to do that. The individual becomes self-critical or self-harming, and in doing so takes an active role, while still hoping to satisfy the abuser. The need to maintain some kind of connection may also be solved by "identification with the aggressor." Re-enacting unhealthy relationships may be another way to turn passive to active, but with the payoff placed in the future in the form of hoping for a different outcome. Another example of turning passive to active through a substitution is hate or controlling behavior aimed at others by someone who has been on the receiving end of bullying or domination.

In Chapter 6, we'll see an interesting feature of the brain's protective systems where the inner mind is more concerned with eliminating the uncomfortable warning signal than the danger it is predicting. The inner mind often seems more interested in killing the messenger than in protecting itself against the danger. Strategies embodied in EMPs designed to suppress the warning signal include dissociation, avoidance of reminders, and distraction from the dreaded internal signal. Others involve cognitive distortions that change meanings to eliminate perceptions that trigger warning signals. Denial and projection are examples. Some strategies involve using thought or behavior to express the opposite of what is dreaded. For example, a client whose inner mind dreads the possibility of weakness might counteract that perception through a life of bodybuilding.

Those are still not all the strategies the human mind is capable of inventing. Among solutions for difficult problems, symbolic substitution is another common strategy. Physical pain of psychological (or physical) origin can become a substitute for emotional pain. In Chapter 5, I'll suggest that anorexia nervosa often involves control over hunger as a symbolic equivalent to controlling neediness for what I call "primal love," the kind that is vital to the lives of very small children. In this case, controlling eating becomes a strategy for keeping a voracious emotional neediness in check. In many cases, where an unnamed fear grips the inner mind (often driven by a biological hypersensitivity), symbolically equivalent fears of real but unlikely dangers generate desperate efforts to calm the anxiety through avoidance. Examples are agoraphobia and fear of travel by air.

Another category addresses problems that can't be solved. Obsessing appears to be one of the inner mind's built-in strategies for creating the impression of solving a problem when no real solution is possible.

Children first begin to develop a sense of right and wrong around age three. Throughout life, this awareness can generate solutions to real-life problems in the form of seeking justice or evening the score. Experiences of hurt can be mitigated by hope for revenge or for the perpetrator to admit to wrongdoing, ask for forgiveness, or be punished. There is a good deal of research indicating that solutions involving retribution or hate may appear satisfying, but in practice are not helpful. Self-punishment and sacrifice can also be pseudo-solutions to problems of injustice or unfairness.

Another major strategy based on the conscience and its capacity to bring shame is internalizing values such as excessive self-sufficiency in a way that causes shame when neediness threatens to surface. This becomes a self-imposed deterrent. I like to call these "internal electric fences" because they act powerfully to keep the individual away from a natural neediness that, at one time, brought painful consequences.

Important strategies may not be immediately apparent because they become part of one's personality or are buried in habit patterns. These can be justified by rationalizations, and they may even have positive consequences, making them seem purposeful and healthy when there might be a more satisfactory solution. Unless it is apparent to the client that trading these for an alternative is worth the effort and cost, the goal of change may be off-limits to psychotherapy. Such hidden strategies can also lead to serious long-term dissatisfaction in life. A talented worker who justifies never becoming a manager might be an example, where the inner reasons might be deeper than the rationalizations. In such cases, it may be up to the therapist to show the client how the pattern is causing unhappiness and that it can be changed. Then the choice is truly up to the client.

Some important threat mitigating strategies are physiological and influenced by genetics and other chemical factors. Depression seems to involve withdrawing and conserving resources in the face of defeat in ways that may have evolved long before humans appeared. Depressed people experience maladaptive impulses to isolate and ruminate on their failures, further deepening painful conscious emotions. Those coping responses to an inborn tendency may be subject to change with psychotherapy. Similarly, anxiety and panic can be responses to the inner mind having a genetic hypersensitivity to danger. EMPs associated with such an inborn sense of danger may embody a strategy of amplifying conscious fears to match an inner sense of dread. An example is "catastrophizing," making things seem worse than they are. Such strategies may be targets of psychotherapy.

The human brain has been described as the most complex structure in the universe. It's not a surprise that it can soothe its own warning signals using a remarkable number of strategies. Many are effective, but the strategies embodied in the problems we treat are often pseudo-solutions. They consist of ways to modify inner meanings to soften their impact and quiet the perception of danger. We can often do better.

The good news for us therapists is that there are often better solutions to replace EMPs. We'll talk about them later as we move toward treatment, most extensively in Chapter 10. As a preview, the single most important and healthiest alternative is often *acceptance*. Making peace with adverse reality is a skill that adults have and children often seem programmed to avoid. With an empathic witness, pain and loss can be healed by accepting reality. That strategy, when it includes grieving for losses and letting anger dissipate, can be applied to many unsolvable problems, including those that once led to the creation of an EMP.

ENTRENCHMENT MEANS RESISTANCE TO CHANGE

Why, then, don't we grow out of our EMPs? Earlier, I said that resistance to change is a fundamental and universal feature of EMPs. The surface explanation is that we are naturally afraid of change. That is true, but there is a more profound reason behind it. The energy the mind spends on avoiding change is evidence that the mind interprets change as dangerous. In other words, change triggers the same survival circuits and threat-mitigating strategies that produce all EMPs.

To the inner mind, psychotherapy is inherently threatening. When our conscious adult client agrees with us that changing an old EMP is a great idea, the inner mind listens in horror. An internal voice says the equivalent of, "You mean you are going to take away a pattern I've been counting on for survival all these years?" Outside of consciousness, the inner mind then mobilizes a new, survival-oriented adaptation to block change from happening. That is what many therapies call *resistance*, an

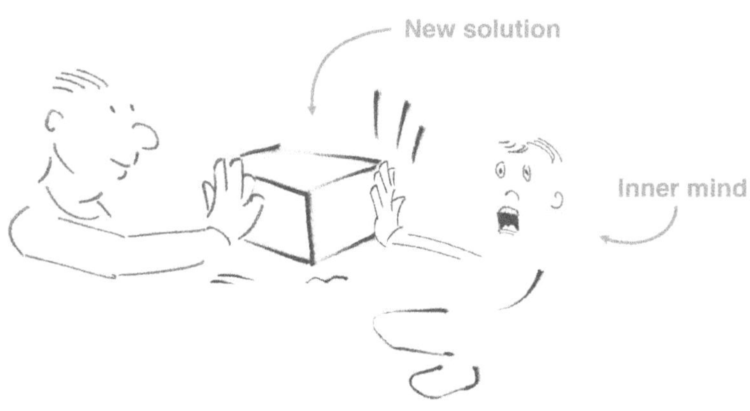

Figure 2.3 Until You Run into Resistance, You're Not Doing Work

involuntary but powerful drive to avoid changes internally perceived as threatening.

An example from healthy child development shows this system in action. Here, too, we see instinctive resistance to an experience that is basically positive but interpreted in a child's mind as a threat. How often do small children say, "I want a drink of water, please!" to stave off having to go to sleep? Their mind appears to appraise the loss of control associated with sleep as a threat and produces a creative response to delay the inevitable. Fortunately, trust in the relationship with caregivers, combined with natural sleepiness, is usually enough to overcome the resistance. Nonetheless, it shows how naturally, instinctively, and cleverly the mind goes to work when it sees a threat.

What is remarkable about this realization is that resistance to change fits precisely into the general definition of EMPs. Strategies for avoiding positive change are *maladaptive*. They impede movement toward health. They are *patterns*, in that they can be identified as such and are likely to be repeated. And, finally, they are *entrenched* in that they take some careful work to overcome. The important implication is that we can use the same tools and techniques in working with this resistance that we do with other kinds of EMPs. If you look back at the earlier list of maladaptive patterns, you will see that one of them is *resistance to healthy change*. When I'm talking specifically about EMPs designed to resist the effects of psychotherapy, I'll sometimes call them *resistance EMPs*.

Arrested Development: An Important Exception

There is one situation where growth can happen without resistance. That is when the inner self knows what it needs in order to restart growth from where it became stuck. It might be a therapist who, at last, is not controlling and trusts the inner self. Maybe that's all that is needed for the young self to go ahead with the exploration and trials needed to gain new skills and experience in life. In such a case, resistance may simply not be present, and progress is fueled by the pleasure inherent in growth. (See "paddling downstream" in Chapter 8.)

Serious Challenges

The most important lesson to take from the mind's strenuous efforts at avoiding change is that the threats that the original EMPs were designed to cope with are not minor. They are serious, even existential in their scale and significance. In adulthood, it may seem hard to understand why an individual would hold onto an obviously maladaptive pattern. When we begin to understand how things looked to the young self at the time an EMP was first invented, it becomes clear that the problems EMPs are designed to solve are very consequential. In addition to entrenchment being a universal feature of EMPs, we can also say that EMPs universally represent coping with threats that are perceived as very serious in nature.

Thinking in terms of EMPs as subunits of pathology is probably a bit unfamiliar. It will turn out to be extremely helpful in navigating the therapeutic space. It is also true that a client can and usually does have a number of EMPs. This is not as worrisome as it might seem. The good news, as we'll see in the next chapter, is that we mostly deal with one of them at a time. The topic of the next chapter is the architecture and organization of multiple EMPs in the same client.

Key Points

- The concept of EMPs captures the essence of the hugely diverse range of problems that psychotherapy is designed to treat.
- *Disorders* are mixtures of psychological and biological symptoms, while EMPs are purely psychological and can be thought of as subunits of pathology treatable in psychotherapy.
- *Entrenched* means the inner mind considers EMPs to be essential protections and finds strategies to resist change.
- Let's flip our view of the mind. The basic mind is the survival-oriented inner mind we share with all mammals. It is the nonconscious one, located subcortically—meaning under the cortex. It is nonverbal and associative in its information processing.
- The other part of the mind is the one we are more familiar with, the conscious, logical one, a fancy add-on given to us by evolution to deal with our hyper-social approach to species survival.
- It seems that evolution set the two minds up to balance each other, but when it comes to motivation and threat processing, the inner mind usually wins.
- EMPs are outdated solutions to problems that, at some point, the inner mind judged so serious that the EMPs became "frozen in time," locked in place, despite there being better ways to respond.
- EMPs use many strategies, but they often add up to ways of avoiding having to face and accept circumstances once deemed so terrible they were unthinkable. The most important adult alternative is *accepting* reality on its terms.

REFERENCES

Ecker, B. (2024). A proposal for the unification of psychotherapeutic action understood as memory modification processes. *Journal of Psychotherapy Integration, 31*(2), 109–125.

Epstein, S. (1994). Integration of the cognitive and the psychodynamic unconscious. *American Psychologist, 49*(8), 709–724.

Hayes, S., & Hofmann, S. (2018). Survival circuits and therapy: From automaticity to the conscious experience of fear and anxiety. *Current Opinion in Behavioral Sciences, 24*, 21–25.

Lane, R. D., & Nadel, L. (2020). *Neuroscience of enduring change: Implications for psychotherapy*. Oxford University Press.

Ledoux, J. (2021). As soon as there was life, there was danger: The deep history of survival behaviours and the shallower history of consciousness. *Philosophical Transactions of the Royal Society B: Biological Sciences, 377*, 20210292.

Panksepp, J., & Biven, L. (2012). *The archaeology of mind: Neuroevolutionary origins of human emotions* (Norton series on interpersonal neurobiology). W. W. Norton & Company.

Wiggins, G. (2020). Creativity, information, and consciousness: The information dynamics of thinking. *Physics of Life Reviews*, 34–35, 1–39.

CHAPTER 3

EMPs Come in Layers

While clients usually have more than one entrenched maladaptive pattern (EMP), the way they fit together is organized and makes sense. In this chapter, we'll develop a bigger picture of how multiple layers of EMPs can coexist simultaneously and how they interact with one another. We'll see how EMPs are organized in layers and how new layers are added when the inner mind predicts the imminent failure of an earlier protection. In addition, we'll use this chapter to go further in showing how EMPs present in the real-life practice of psychotherapy.

EMPs Are Organized Like the Defenses of a Medieval Castle

EMPs are set up like the defenses of a medieval castle. In the Middle Ages, enemies first encountered a hill, then a moat, then an outer wall. Finally, they'd reach the inner sanctum, the final barrier. Like castles, the mind's protections are constructed starting with the innermost *keep*, where we find the thickest walls and most impenetrable protection. Outer walls and perimeters are built in successive layers.

Psychotherapy takes the same course as capturing a castle, starting with the outer defenses. This usually means we start with the EMP that is least defended, most recent, and most accessible. Here are two examples showing both the complexity of real-world psychotherapy, and how complexity can be approached, one EMP at a time.

Panic attacks are a typical example. They often come with no warning, as happened to a client named John, a 34-year-old construction supervisor. To all appearances, he seemed to be riding high in his life and career. In close succession, he received a promotion and learned

DOI: 10.4324/9781003619659-4

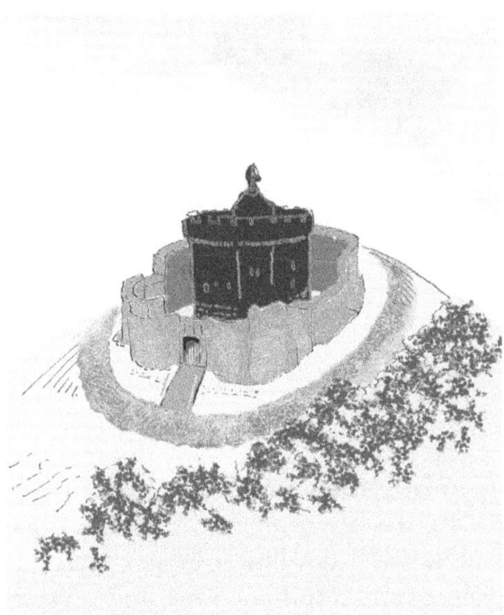

Figure 3.1 Layered Protections

that his wife was pregnant with their first child. Then, out of nowhere, he has a panic attack at work and is taken to the emergency room. He is referred for therapy. His new therapist soon discovers that he had a tough background and had learned always to be self-sufficient and never depend on anyone.

She realizes that his deepest and earliest layer of EMP is to avoid any kind of dependence. In his childhood, neediness would only bring disappointment and punishment. On the other hand, recent events in his life, though positive, have increased his natural and healthy need for support. Tension between his inner mind's neediness and its equally energetic rejection of any kind of help stretches him to the breaking point. His inner mind detects that something has to give, and launches a new EMP, the panic attack. That gives short-term relief by removing him from his job. On the other hand, he is referred for therapy, where the promise of support further inflames his inner neediness, which, in turn, threatens his cherished self-sufficiency. His inner mind's first reaction is to launch yet another EMP. This one is a protective rationalization that pops into his consciousness. He tells the therapist that he "won't need much help" and will "only stay for one session."

This newest layer of EMP is in the category of resistance to therapy. It is modeled on the previous one, prohibiting him from accepting help. This time, however, his inner mind rightly senses that therapy could bring relief and emotional support. That would threaten his stability by whetting his appetite for yet more support, and that could overwhelm him. Faced with colliding needs, his inner mind appraises an insoluble problem and shows signs of maximum stress, which could lead to more panic attacks. The urgent priority is to bring some calm amid conflicting needs.

The therapist starts with the most superficial of the EMPs, resistance to therapy. She has learned that one of John's strengths is following procedures. Creatively, she explains that therapy is a procedure required for people with panic attacks and will necessitate some additional sessions. Reluctantly, with the encouragement of his wife, he accepts the sessions, sensing the therapist's verbal and nonverbal cues that he could trust her not to make him too dependent and that she would help him strengthen his ability to soldier on at work as well as in his role as a new father.

The therapist's strategy of emphasizing therapy as a routine procedure may be a bit manipulative, though not dishonest. She knows that his excessive self-sufficiency is an EMP based on a value system, and those are particularly resistant to change. The EMP that overvalues self-sufficiency is so deeply internalized, it will have to come later in treatment. First, he'll need positive experiences of therapy, presented as a necessary procedure.

What Triggers the Creation of EMPs?

The trigger for the creation of the first and deepest layer of EMP is a serious, even existential challenge to the individual. For John, it was the pain he experienced as a small boy when seeking the support and attention he naturally needed. We have also seen that, while the challenges faced by humans tend to be similar, each person's experience and their solutions are uniquely individual.

Even when biology is prominent, for example with people who are genetically prone to anxiety, each one's adaptation to an inner sense of danger is unique. One client might obsess over fears of a terrible health condition but be able to fly in airplanes, while another is terrified of air travel, but never thinks about cancer. In all cases, our curiosity should lead us beyond the surface concern into the deeper and more personal one behind it. "What, exactly, are you afraid of in taking a plane?" Maybe the fear is the moment of realizing that the plane is going down, or it might be feelings about losing connections with loved ones. Behind the outward symptoms, we will find unique emotional concerns. Accurate empathy requires going as far as possible to understand the deepest dread. That will turn out to be vital when it comes to supporting change.

EMPs Can Be Complicated

Early in his life, George was terrorized by his father's rigid, religious, by-the-book righteousness. His original EMP was to internalize his father's morality and vow always to be good. This worked well as he joined Boy Scouts, attended church, and grew up to enter an apparently healthy, high-functioning adolescence. His avoidance of sex did not seem unusual and did not cause much stress. He had a few arguments with his father but remained loyal to the moral principles.

In college, the culture, as well as his inner drive to join the adult world, led him to alcohol and sex, which he had previously avoided. Tension built between his inner instinct to become an adult and his rigid morality. A new layer of EMP was somehow to do both: follow his father's morality *and* grow into a happy adult. It was doomed to fail. One day, he attended a party with a friend, who became drunk but wanted to drive home. George couldn't muster the clarity to take away the keys but got in the car to accompany his drunk friend. The friend crashed, and the client went into a moral tailspin. He left school, went to confession, and temporarily turned away from his first love as well as alcohol. His inner mind had re-evaluated his newfound freedom and decided it had been a terrible mistake. He retreated to his original adaptation.

Gradually the newer EMP, to adopt both conflicting goals, returned, but in a new form. Now it consisted in keeping up an appearance of adulthood while accepting an arrested maturation beyond college. He lived out an uneasy compromise between his dour conscience and his healthy desire to grow. He married and had children but dropped out of graduate school and never developed a career. His wife reluctantly supported him, while his friends and neighbors assumed he was a high-functioning, normal family man. As time passed, he realized that life was finite and that the one he was living was not at all the one he wanted.

In therapy, he gradually came to understand that he would have to break free from his EMP compromise to find his own adult morality and restart his path to an adult career. Against strong internal resistance, he struggled toward growth in both areas.

This case exemplifies both how the failure of one EMP can trigger the formation of a new one, and how an EMP can be an adaptation to cope with two competing threats, in this case, the threat of immorality versus the threat of failure to grow up.

Do We Have to Know About All Layers?

Fortunately, the answer is no, we don't have to know about all the EMPs. Often, one layer alone will be apparent, and that is the one we start with. If there is a choice, we usually work with the one that is most readily accessible. We also want to help the client see results, which may involve prioritizing an EMP that will lead to symptom resolution or increased satisfaction in life. Finding successes along the way, when possible, is fortunate in that it helps maintain the client's level of hope and motivation to keep up with the work. As we make progress on one layer, others beneath it will emerge and become accessible for change. Sometimes we can see far ahead, but just as often it is like traveling in thick fog, where we can only see what is right in front of us, and not much beyond. Fortunately, we don't have to have a full hypothesis about a layer until we are ready to engage in working with it.

In George's case, a surprise EMP only became apparent far into his treatment. He seemed intent on finding and building his adult career, but as the therapy progressed, results were glacially slow in coming. He also seemed to relate to me as an authority more than a support and helper. What gradually became apparent was that his father had also taught him, at any cost, to hide anything negative about the family. His EMP was to avoid letting his therapist see the magnitude of his difficulty. As his being stuck became undeniable, he began to share how he would make plans for the day, then spend hours distracting himself, while feeling bad about his lack of accomplishment. As he shared his struggle, he opened a healthy door and let me in where I could seek a new level of accurate empathy. That allowed new energy to begin to flow, and with it progress in seeking an adult life and career.

EMPs Can Present Themselves in Three Different Ways

While discussing how EMPs manifest themselves, it is helpful to distinguish between three quite distinct ways EMPs can present in sessions. Each one requires a different approach and different objectives. They are based on the extent to which the client's inner emotions are causing *affect* to be present in the room. Here is some practical guideance.

WHEN AFFECT IS IMMEDIATELY PRESENT

Not infrequently, clients arrive in a state of intense emotion. At other times, emotions bloom within the session. Either way, their emergence is a wonderful opportunity for further accurate empathy. Here are some thoughts about how to handle the situation.

Of course, the first thing is to assess whether there is any real danger and raise the level of care, if required, by bringing in additional resources.

Assuming there is no immediate danger, the next goal is to bring the situation within a workable window of intensity. The first question is whether the client is "dysregulated," meaning so overcome with emotion that they are no longer in control. There are many tools for helping, but most of them capture elements from the original soothing experience that almost all of us have had. What do mothers do for children who are dysregulated? They make physical contact, stay very present, use a quiet, soothing tone of voice, and listen. As therapists, physical contact is usually not appropriate, but our presence is enough. This powerful use of the relationship is one of our best tools and should never be forgotten. Here, it is especially important to recall that our *ears* do the hard work, not our mouths. Active attempts to calm the client are usually interpreted by the client's inner mind as motivated by the therapist's need for calm, rather than the client's need to be understood.

In the meantime, science, augmented by openness to Eastern practices, has incorporated techniques like mindfulness and controlled breathing to activate the calming parasympathetic branch of the autonomic nervous system. With practice, clients learn breathing techniques and other ways to self-soothe. Note that this requires some preparation. Introducing physical techniques in the middle of dysregulation could break the emotional connection. As in childhood, an emotional presence is the first and most important ingredient. The therapist's calm presence is a powerful, experiential way to communicate a more mindful attitude. We don't always need words, and often the experience of having a calm witness is more communicative anyway.

As we begin to seek understanding, a first phase requires being quiet, listening, and observing. Asking questions too early disrupts the flow of emotion from the inner mind and can signal impatience on the part of the listener. In an unhurried way, we then begin to seek accurate empathy. That might mean continuing simply to listen, or it might involve waiting, then softly and gently asking a question or two. The dysregulation will almost always abate, and real communication will begin, where the client is now sharing what is upsetting, and we are positioned to begin building our understanding.

The Art of the Question

Questions are an important way (in addition to listening) to gain understanding. The most challenging question is silence, at least in a context where the client has been instructed to say whatever comes to mind. Silence puts the inner mind into some turmoil, not knowing what to reveal and what to hide, or how you will react. From there, any words you put in a question will narrow the field from the infinite range demanded by silence. Narrowing is soothing because the question becomes easier to answer until it gets too narrow. Too narrow results in the kind of questions a district attorneys asks, "Did you or did you not..." DAs want to box the witness in. Being boxed in creates unnecessary discomfort for the client, and that's not at all what we want in therapy. So, for every client, there is a mid-ground between too open and too narrow.

People who are more intellectual can handle abstract questions without necessarily becoming *too* intellectual: "Tell me about the course of your life so far." Professor Mallory could respond to that question and would welcome the chance to share his already extensive thoughtfulness. John, who appreciates procedural approaches, is less intellectual and wouldn't know what we are looking for. He would do better with concrete questions like, "Then what did you do?"

If you want to hear about emotions, ask for facts. "How did you react to that?" If you ask directly, "How did you feel?" your question is likely to be interpreted as "What abnormal feeling did you have?" It will be misinterpreted as wanting to apply a label or to find something pathological. Not good.

So, by asking a question, we are creating a container big enough to hold what we want while leaving the client freedom to fill it in their own way, whatever that may be.

Remember that a question is like an unfinished story. It will niggle the client's inner mind until the answer comes. The answer may arrive within seconds, minutes, or not, and is likely to be communicated in a way you may not expect or even notice. So, it helps to remember what has been asked and what questions are still on the table. Those are the blanks that your curiosity, as well as the client's, will be eager to fill in.

Working with an Emotionally Charged Experience

As we begin to make progress toward understanding, we begin in earnest to help the client use our accurate empathy to process an emotionally charged experience.

Let's not forget reality. Maybe the client has just learned about a life circumstance that has no solution or one that demands action. As human beings, we know that a real emergency needs to take precedence over the goals of psychotherapy. Maybe our role is to help with emotional regulation so the client can access the resources needed to deal with a real-life challenge.

Having clarified that no immediate action need be taken, our mission is then to seek accurate empathy. Simply doing that will help the client process their emotions. Our quietness and patience are demonstrations of our respect for the intensity of feeling and our interest in understanding. Next, we hope the client will begin to tell us what is going on. This can require some minimal prompts, but the less we say, the freer the client may feel to tell us what they are experiencing, which reveals aspects we might not have known to ask about.

When the emotion is in proportion to reality, there may not be an EMP in play. The client's response may be a healthy reaction. We may simply be witnessing a normal emotional response to a difficult event. If so, our job is still to be a compassionate witness. It is a valid use of time to use our understanding to help soothe the client as one human to another. On the other hand, when the emotion is out of proportion and larger than one might expect, that is a likely indication that an EMP has been activated.

Why Oversized Emotions Suggest an EMP and What to Do

When our natural sense says the emotion is out of proportion to reality, our curiosity should lead us to wonder why. It usually means a circumstance is being experienced by a part of the inner mind that got stuck earlier in life. Younger children, and even young adults, experience stronger feelings. As we mature, the cerebral cortex gradually becomes more dominant, and intense feelings are suppressed. When the emotions are more intense than we might expect, it usually means the circumstances are being evaluated by a part of the inner mind that is frozen in time at a point where bigger emotion *is indeed* appropriate to the circumstances. As we understand the past origin of the emotion, we will be able to acknowledge the intensity of feeling and, as we seek accurate empathy, come to understand the emotion from the point of view of the young inner self that is experiencing it today.

Beginning to understand the full context surrounding an emotion is a good start to healing or processing the emotion. Healing happens when the inner self sees an old, intense, and self-absorbed experience in a new light; when the inner self is able to see the event through the eyes of the therapist witness. The calm embodied by the therapist puts the experience in a larger perspective. That is mindfulness. When the change becomes permanent, we'll learn that memory reconsolidation is how the inner transformation has taken place.

To be complete, there is a phenomenon where even intense emotions may not be the authentic kind for this type of processing. As clarified in emotion focused therapy (Aledort, 1999), *instrumental emotions* are used to control or manipulate another person. In addition, *secondary emotions* can cover up a more threatening, but authentic, emotion. An example of the latter is anger used by the inner mind to cover up sadness. When these alternative forms of emotion are present, seeking accurate empathy will not give immediate relief but can lead to identification of a hidden EMP in which those emotions serve a protective purpose. Those EMPs are among the less visible ones to be described in the third section below.

When emotions are immediately present in the room, our goal is to make use of the opportunity to seek accurate empathy and allow it to transform the experience. Our warm but calm presence sends powerful regulating messages, while our persistent interest invites the client to let us further into their inner world and fulfill conditions for transformative change, that is, healing.

WHEN AFFECT IS NEAR BUT NOT YET PRESENT

When emotions are near, but not yet present or "in the room," the client does not show significant affect, but we can sense that hot issues are near. Our job, then, is to coax the emotion into the room.

How do we know there is emotion nearby? Perhaps it is a slight touch of affect or a certain intensity in the client's narrative. Our curiosity and natural instincts usually tell us there is something almost ready to come to light. If so, then the question for the therapist is, "What is blocking its expression?" Here is a useful decision tree to help in monitoring and responding to the flow of information when emotion is near but not yet fully present.

The Three-Step Dance

As long as the flow of information is moving along and you are learning new things about the client, then do nothing but listen, and, at most, indicate that you are following what they're saying. If the flow of fresh insight slows or stops, here are three steps to take. I call it the three-step dance.

A. **The nudge:** When the flow of new information slows or stops, then give a mild indication that you expect more. I call this a nudge. It might be a question, but in the direction the conversation is going. "Could you give me an example?" or "I'd like to hear a bit more about that." If this gets the client moving again, giving you fresh details, then no further action is needed. No EMP was blocking the communication. The nudge is a test, and the results are indicated by the response. If the nudge fails to get you moving again, it means there is a significant blockage, and behind it, there is almost certainly an EMP.
B. **Metacommunication:** When the nudge test indicates a real blockage, it means the subject of the conversation has changed. Now it's about discomfort regarding what would have been revealed. The client's inner mind is now focused on something threatening about the conversation. Because the true subject has changed, it will not feel jarring or disruptive to shift the focus to the conversation itself. A term for this new subject is *metacommunication*, that is, talking *about the communication*. Specifically, we want to address the difficulty the client is having sharing emotional content that is near, but not yet in the room. We need to be direct. Here is a place where beginners often err by trying to circumvent the blockage or by ignoring it. Humans are very sensitive and wary of any attempt to sneak around their defenses. It also won't work to ignore the problem; that will leave the client feeling you are not tuned in. So, we put the new problem into words: "It seems like this is hard for you. Take your time. Maybe you could start by telling me about…" This is metacommunication. There is no formula, and social instincts are still our best teachers about what will help the client to overcome an inner reluctance and reveal something less than comfortable.
C. **Strategic retreat:** Metacommunication is a test, too. If it doesn't work to overcome the blockage, it means that, for the present, the barrier is too high. If so, it is critical to say out loud that you will let go for now, but keep the question open as long as needed. After retreating, it is essential not to forget because the inner mind will interpret that as not caring. "This seems like a tender subject. It's ok to leave it for now. We'll come back to it when the time is right."

These strategies, plus tact and thoughtful interest, will keep the dialogue progressing toward increasing revelation. Accurate empathy will build and bring affect closer to the room. Until then, understanding the EMP layers standing in the way has become the new and important topic in therapy.

WHEN THE AFFECT IS FAR AWAY

In this last situation, the lack of affect is an indication that an EMP is more solidly in place, keeping nonconscious emotion well under control and hidden. Maybe it looks like a personality trait, or maybe its functioning is so smooth that it has not yet been noticed. Since EMPs are, by definition, maladaptive, they have a negative effect on the person's life. It may help to ask oneself if there is some client characteristic that, if changed, might lead to a more satisfactory life experience.

Linda was appreciated and valued because she was always ready to help. She would freely give her time and even money, though she scarcely had enough for herself. She had many friends who depended on her. She also indulged her daughter beyond a level that was reasonable. Only occasionally, circumstances would result in her withholding. Every time she did so, there was a good reason, but her daughter, in particular, would feel the shock, as she always expected to come first. At these times, there would be friction, smoothed over by more indulgence. As this went on from year to year, Linda couldn't understand why she had trouble controlling her use of alcohol and why she was always working extra hours to fill a hole in her budget.

Linda's own mother had been intensely narcissistic and taught Linda from early in life that her duty was first to support her mother's self-esteem. Linda understood that being a model daughter was the only way to support her mother's self-image as "the best." Doing so gave Linda the nonconscious hope that her devotion would someday enable her mother to love her. In adulthood, she continued the pattern of giving too much to others, including her daughter. The hidden costs were a constant need filled by drinking, as well as damage to her daughter's sense of how to receive real love.

To friends and family, Linda seemed like a fine and generous person with a few odd quirks, like arguing with her daughter and sometimes drinking too much.

The job of a therapist goes beyond simply noting such quirks or personality traits to being curious about the reasons for their existence. When we follow our curiosity to learn why, we begin to uncover hidden EMPs. When we think we have found one, the first task is to ask ourselves if there is a link between the EMP and the problem that brought the client to therapy. In Linda's case, it was the link between her drinking and a constant sense of emptiness, caused by giving too much. Having made the connection between the maladaptive characteristic with its consequences, we can move toward making that EMP the focus of the work. That's how we start the slow process of eventually bringing deeply hidden affects like Linda's feeling of need and emptiness into the room.

When will that happen? It will when the client begins to change behavior. If Linda stops drinking, anger and resentment will surface. If she takes better care of herself, guilt and shame will come to the fore. Each of her maladaptive behaviors, giving and drinking, serves to keep the other in balance, so changing one is likely to cause the other to get out of control. We'll need to monitor both.

When Linda begins to take better care of herself and drink less, she will experience a lot of affect. Understanding this and helping Linda anticipate her feeling reactions will help greatly with motivation and trust in the process. She may also find that old friends who took advantage of her begin to distance themelves, while new, healthier friends are attracted to her. It may even start her daughter on a path to looking more closely at herself.

It's worth noting that approaching Linda's drinking as the only problem, without an appreciation of the underlying EMP, would probably not work out well. In fact, while alcohol addiction can be heavily genetic and a problem in itself, in this case, treating it as the only problem would be bad therapy. Its role in self-medicating her inner neediness will not go away. Success at abstinence without dealing with her excessive generosity would unbalance her emotional system, a lot like when one person suddenly gets off the teeter-totter. Her inner mind would find a way to compensate for her unmet need, but it would probably not be a good one.

For better or worse, not all clients are motivated to make changes to this kind of hidden EMP. Only when we can agree to target the EMP will it become a subject of the therapy. If it is more of an incidental finding, then the job of showing how change might be beneficial will be challenging. We'll have to do a good job of connecting the EMP with real suffering, missing out on something desirable, or both. The best source of motivation is the client's own pain, lack of satisfaction, or vision of a better life. We can only go so far in promoting efforts to change this kind of EMP.

In this chapter, we have begun to paint an overall picture of how layers of EMPs can reduce health and satisfaction in life. In the next chapter, we will look more closely at the inner selves that are the authors of all EMPs.

Key Points

- Unlike the mixtures of symptoms that make up disorders, EMPs are self-contained subunits of pathology designed to solve problems the inner mind once experienced as very serious.
- Each client is likely to have multiple layers of EMPs, organized like the defenses of a medieval castle.
- What triggers the creation of a new EMP is the inner mind's prediction that an existing layer is going to fail.
- Fortunately, we don't have to understand all the layers to work with the one or two that are most accessible and important in improving life.
- Affects such as tears or tone of voice are automatic bodily signs of activation in the inner mind, our best indicators that it has detected a threat.
- When affect is present in the room, we need to listen quietly, then seek accurate empathy.
- When affect is near, but not present, we need to invite it to come closer using a three-step dance.
- Step 1 is noticing a slowing in the flow of information and giving a nudge to determine if it is a sign of an emotional blockage.
- Step 2 is using metacommunication to focus on the blockage itself.
- Step 3 is to determine whether the blockage is too big for now and must be put off for later, but not forgotten.
- When affect is far away and not accessible, it probably means that it is made of EMPs that are embodied in habits and personality traits.

REFERENCE

Aledort, S. (1999). Working with emotions in psychotherapy. *The Journal of Psychotherapy Practice and Research, 8*, 249–250.

CHAPTER 4

Inner Selves, the Authors of EMPs

In this chapter, we pick up on the thread started in Chapter 2 where we discussed flipping our view of the mind. At that time, we introduced the idea that an instinctive inner mind, similar to those of other mammals and dedicated to the survival of the species, is our basic equipment for knowing how to get along in the world. We viewed the inner mind as primary, with powerful and extensive tools for exerting influence on our conscious decision-making through automatic thoughts, feelings, and impulses. In contrast, we viewed the conscious mind as a "fancy add-on" that gives us humans advantages as well as *some* ability to edit and filter the survival-oriented products of our inner mind.

The theme of this chapter is that the inner mind and its component selves are the first authors of the EMPs that psychotherapy is designed to treat. Having an understanding and appreciation of these inner selves will help us greatly in working with them and the EMPs they produce.

WHY THINK OF THE INNER MIND AS A SELF?

Under healthy conditions, the inner mind is a seamless partner with our healthy conscious mind. The two complement each other, even as they sometimes disagree. A good example is curiosity. Belonging to the inner mind, curiosity operates largely outside of consciousness, where it works tirelessly to find holes in our knowledge and prompts our consciousness to wonder about the answers. Curiosity is the source of our love for stories and our endless fascination with how they end. And questions are powerful because they trigger a desire for the satisfaction of knowing the end result, the answer. A question is a story without an end. It sets both minds, ours and the client's, on a quest, seeking the missing piece. It is

DOI: 10.4324/9781003619659-5

the inner mind that keeps working as we sleep and often serves up the answer in the morning when we least expect it.

How an Inner Self Is the Inventor of Every EMP

What happens in the inner mind when there is no answer? And, more importantly for us, what if the problem is so severe that it threatens our very existence? We can answer those questions by looking at what happens in early development when the inner mind solves a problem as best it can, then holds tightly to that answer. At that point, a part of the inner mind becomes frozen in time. When those frozen solutions and plans appear in adulthood, we see them as purposeful, as if that part of the mind had become an agent in itself. Because it is frozen in time, it has become insulated, disassociated from the rest of the inner mind as well as from consciousness. For the sake of survival, this self remains driven to impose its solution. That is how EMPs work. They are, in effect, carried by an inner self and persist indefinitely until something powerful changes them.

What is the evidence for this origin story? The persistence of EMPs in spite of their heavy cost supports their existence and separateness from the rest of the client's functioning. The fact that they can be triggered by events in adult life, such as the birth of a child or a loss, suggests that they can persist in some form behind the scenes. They appear sometimes later in life, apparently set in motion by the sense that life is finite, and it is high time to complete the plan, further suggesting that an inner self has remained vigilant, waiting for the time to be ripe.

This is where experience gained from the psychodynamic point of view helps sharpen and test ways to make sense of information processing that goes on outside of consciousness. When accurate empathy brings us close to a true understanding, clients report that some thoughts resonate, while those that miss the mark don't. More importantly, as therapy succeeds in unraveling an EMP, we witness time and time again that affects, formerly suppressed by the EMP, appear on the surface as expected. In this way, every case is a research project with testable hypotheses and specific individual results. They are not statistical because no two cases are the same, but when our hypotheses are sharp and clear, the results can give a definitive answer, positive or negative.

When we add the overall knowledge that the inner mind is an organ devoted to survival, and when we understand that its information processing is much like the thinking of a child, then formulations like those in the cases of John and Anna not only make good sense but give us the waypoints and sightings we need to navigate these otherwise mysterious waters.

Personification

The reason thinking of the inner self as a person works so well is that EMPs are real solutions, invented by the self while facing a very serious, even existential problem. Now, in therapy, the solution is no longer ideal, but the self who created it is frozen in time and remains desperately motivated to apply the original solution. Freud called this a fixation. The client, often at a young age, invents the best solution possible with the resources available. Since that solution is guarding against disaster, it is held tightly and rigidly. The author of the problem is fixated, holding the solution as if it stood between life and death. This means the inner self, the author of that solution, operates with intense purposefulness and determination, not as an abstract concept, but like a person fighting for their life. Understanding this is enormously helpful to us therapists because we are no longer surprised by the deeply rooted and driven quality of EMPs. With that understanding, we are far better prepared to work with a frightened young self who needs to let go and try something new.

To do such work, I argue in this chapter that it is time to go beyond what has often been considered dispassionate and scientific. It is quite possible that this independent self consists only of a set of rules for how the person should respond and pattern matching to determine their application. However, the metaphor of a separate being is highly useful and faithful to observation in portraying how threat processing systems include purpose, will, plans, and the motivation to see them carried out.

I would suggest that personifying the source of EMPs as an inner self is actually more accurate than trying to be scientific by viewing the phenomenon in an impersonal way. A more "scientific" view of irrational thoughts as cognitive distortions fails to recognize their purposefulness and persistence. EMPs include not only perceptions and behaviors, but strong motivation, persistence over time, and monitoring of their implementation and success or failure. The latter is evidenced by instantaneous feelings of elation and depression depending on whether the solution is going to plan. Those characteristics are far more completely and accurately captured by the metaphor of an active inner self than by dry descriptions of deviation from what is considered "normal."

In case there is a need for further support of the idea of personifying the authors of EMPs, the idea is backed by research from internal family systems therapy. Founded by Richard Schwartz on the idea of inner selves as participants in therapy, proponents have done extensive research (Schwartz, 2013). And, by the way, they give memorably descriptive names to inner selves such as "managers," "exiles," and "firefighters."

To summarize, thinking in terms of an inner self as the author of every EMP is, in many ways, more truthful than viewing nonconsciously driven behavior impersonally as a manifestation of faulty beliefs and perceptions. Viewing the source of such patterns as an inner person brings the EMP to life. Technically, it respects the otherwise neglected dimensions of motivation, planning, and purposefulness, strongly characteristic of EMPs, and regularly embodied in their outer expression.

THE EVOLUTIONARY BIOLOGY OF THE INNER SELF

The late Jaak Panksepp and Lucy Biven (2012) describe the origins of our inner emotional mind as follows:

> *"As far as we know right now, primal emotional systems evolved a very long time ago and that at a basic emotional and motivational level, all mammals are more similar than they are different."*

What Panksepp, Le Doux, and by now, many others have studied is a group of brain structures located underneath the cerebral cortex and closely analogous to those of other mammals. Those structures include the amygdala, hippocampus, cingulate gyrus, and more. Technically, we can call them subcortical; informally, they are often referred to as limbic, referring to their role in the origin of emotions.

In particular, much of Panksepp's work has consisted of experiments in which analogous subcortical areas are experimentally activated in humans in parallel to other mammals. With activation of analogous brain structures, humans report powerful emotional experiences, while the animals show bodily responses intuitively recognizable as similar to ours in emotional content.

As an example, we might be getting too close to our dog while she is eating from her dish. She growls, and we interpret her response as showing a bit of irritation, if not anger. Neurophysiologists such as Ledoux might argue that we can't know what the dog feels since dogs don't seem to have our kind of consciousness. That is hard to deny, but Panksepp would point out that in the dog's brain the same structures are activated that are active in humans who are subjectively feeling threatened. Like the lay observer, Panksepp would tend to conclude that the dog is, in all likelihood, experiencing something we could call anger. So far, the argument seems more a matter of language than anything else, since nobody knows what animals, lacking speech, subjectively feel. In this context, it is worth considering that, given a baby's similar lack of words, our conjecture about animal experiences of emotion is no more or less valid than our universal willingness to name what a baby is "feeling."

What makes humans different is that our consciousness can make connections and give meaning to events in ways that probably go well beyond what other mammals can. What is not entirely clear is how much the firing of the amygdala and other deep structures is transmitted directly to consciousness. What scientists agree on is that conscious feelings are constructed, with some input from the subcortical mind as well as additional elements such as past experience, translation into words, and additional associations. Thus, we should not think of activity in the subcortical mind as identical to conscious feelings. They are related, but not the same. Perhaps the best way to express the relationship is that subcortical, limbic structures are able to produce *emotional precursors* or *proto-emotions.*

Nonconscious Emotions

It will be apparent later that the role of nonconscious proto-emotions is more fundamental than their causing bodily affects and conscious feelings. They represent the final step in triggering the activation and launching of complete EMPs. The critical implication is that if the neural activation we are thinking of as an emotional precursor does not take place, then there will be no EMP. That makes them important targets for psychotherapy.

The components of EMP responses made up of bodily affects and conscious feelings are extremely important because of their influence on conscious experience and what they tell us as therapists. I use the word *feelings* to mean those conscious states we recognize as emotion. Affects, in contrast, are the earliest involuntary bodily responses triggered by nonconscious subcortical emotions. When present, affects give us a window into what is going on in the subcortical mind. Affects and conscious feelings add up to those in-session emotions that have been shown to correlate with success in therapy (Whelton, 2004). Unfortunately, to date, there is no clear agreement about what to call nonconscous emotional signals. For our purposes, because they are not conscious and because they are emotional, I'll call them *nonconscious emotions.*

Because our grasp of nonconscious emotions is indirect, we do need to be careful when drawing conclusions about just what is happening in the subcortical mind. When we observe bodily affects, appearing automatically as the first responses to nonconscious emotion, our inborn capacity for empathy indicates their basic character. Furthermore, in therapy, clients can often verbalize what led to an affective response. When we share a description of what we think might be going on beneath our client's consciousness, we often get a clear response indicating that our version is off the mark or that it "resonates" with something inside them. For myself, and many other therapists, client reports, as well as such resonance, have been invaluable tools for clarifying inner mental contents and nonconscious emotions. As indicated earlier, this leads to hypotheses, which can be tested by observing what happens as we continue to conduct the therapy.

How do we handle the uncertainty? We hold our hypotheses with a light touch. When they are corroborated by other observations, and especially when they lead to change, we tend to think of them as *probably confirmed*.

In addition to the clinical usefulness of the concept of nonconscious emotions, there is considerable experimental science to verify their existence. Their neural equivalents can be confirmed in the laboratory. Furthermore, the same neural activations can be measured in the complete absence of conscious awareness. When an emotionally charged image is shown for such a short time that it doesn't register consciously, changes have regularly been measured showing that an emotional response has nonetheless been generated. Thus, research confirms the existence of emotion in the complete absence of consciousness (Smith & Lane, 2016).

Communication with Inner Selves

To help you picture the operation of the inner mind and how to communicate with it, let's look at some examples from outside the field of psychotherapy. Examples of communicating with the inner, basic mind of a mammal are seen in the television show *The Dog Whisperer* with Cesar Milan. There, Milan shows dog owners how to understand their dog's responses and, in doing so, helps them know how to approach what had seemed like an impasse. A gentle nudge with his foot tells the dog he is the boss and that the dog can let go and follow, rather than needing to be the alpha dog and take responsibility for the safety of the pack. Milan does so in a way that leaves the dog acting happy and relaxed. As stated above, subcortical components of the dog's mind that generate patterns of response are quite close to those subcortical parts of the human mind responsible for ensuring safety. A significant aspect of psychotherapy is communicating in similarly nonverbal ways with the client's inner mind. For example, our calm in the face of the client's upset is an important nonverbal communication that says, "It's going to be alright."

In a human example, Supernanny, the star of another TV show, comes into a family where parents have lost control of the household and the children. With little or no participation of the children's rational minds, they become happy, motivated, and energized as never before. As they do so, the parents begin to understand their leadership role in managing the instinctive responses of the children. We see how the children's responses get stuck in patterns that lead to unhappiness for the whole family. We also witness how rapidly and dramatically they change when Supernanny, and later the parents, show understanding, firmness, and consistency.

Readiness to picture an inner self with nonconscious emotion, motivation, plans, and purposefulness gives us the ability to think of goings-on in the subcortical brain that are not so different from a dog or a child, actively predicting threats and generating adaptations. In these situations, it is not as much our intellectual knowledge as it is our intuitive understanding that sets empathy in motion and shows us how to relate to and communicate with the inner author of an EMP. While it may feel strange, the truth is that, compared with ideas we exchange with the conscious adult client, communication with an inner self is as much, if not more, responsible for the lasting changes that come out of psychotherapy. The subcortical inner mind does not use words in its information processing. Even the positive effects of our words are due to their being translated into nonverbal terms as they are passed down from consciousness to subcortical areas where nonverbal meaning is the native langage.

Neurophysiology isn't the only place where scientific thinkers have noticed the inner mind. In the next section, the discussion is related to the work of cognitive researchers as well as Daniel Kahneman, who won a Nobel Prize for describing how humans, contrary to the previous assumptions of economists, do not always make rational economic decisions, and that their irrationality comes from an inner mind (Kahneman, 2011).

THE SCIENCE OF SYSTEM 1 AND SYSTEM 2

When an unexpected thread of science turns up that confirms one's working hypothesis, it tends to give additional confidence. That's what happened for me when I learned that cognitive science was also talking about an inner mind different from the conscious one. For some time now, cognitive scientists have been looking at how people make decisions. They realized that, not infrequently, and as described by Freud, something outside of consciousness interferes with logical decision-making. That spawned the dual-process view of mind.

Cognitive science coined the terms *System 1* and *System 2*, respectively, to describe and contrast the nonconscious mode compared to the more familiar conscious one. These coincide with what I have been calling the inner mind, as opposed to consciousness. Joseph Evans (2003), a pioneer in the area, described System 1 as the nonconscious, autonomous, and protective component of a dual-process theory of mental information processing. Not long after, Daniel Kahneman popularized the phrase "thinking fast," to describe System 1 and compared it to "thinking slow," the conscious, logical, and somewhat less bias-prone form of thinking. The field of cognitive science has continued to study the differences between these modes of information processing, but has, so far, shown only modest interest in the richness of System 1 beyond its ability to give quick-and-dirty answers. For myself, and Richard Lane, MD, PhD (personal communication), the distinction between the two is highly valuable in understanding the differences between nonconscious information processing and the conscious kind that is necessarily more familiar. As therapists, we want to become experts in understanding and communicating with the inner mind in its own terms.

Inner Mind Versus Conscious Mind: How Distinct Are They?

Interestingly, cognitive science has some objections to the dual-process view of mind (Da Silva, 2023). In contrast to those who see the two processes as highly distinct, others have argued that the two are often too closely entangled to separate them, and the dividing line can't be cleanly defined. We have already made an observation that offers a path to resolving these differences.

In the previous chapter, we discussed how the inner mind, faced with a serious problem, tends to become frozen in time and separate from the rest of the mind as it holds tightly to its solution to a major problem. Entrenchment means the inner mind mobilizes active responses to defend its protective strategy from being changed. It's as if life depended on keeping it the same. This is where the inner mind turns away from its partner, the conscious one, and begins to function separately and independently, often in opposition to conscious desire. Thus, in health, the two minds operate in close partnership, while the presence of an EMP causes their functioning to become separate and distinct.

In fact, we can join with cognitive scientists and broaden our perspective on human irrationality when we notice that the inner mind's separateness and independence live on a spectrum. The earlier and more life-threatening the problem behind an EMP, the more rigid and separate is the functioning of the inner self. Some of the most rigid and entrenched EMPs, such as attachment styles and personality disorders, come from early in development when insoluble problems in life are appraised more as existential, life–death challenges. EMPs created later and on the spot, like the ones that defend against change in therapy, are often more easily let go.

Along similar, but positive lines, it appears that with healthier early development, a deep-seated optimism, sometimes called *basic trust*, can become internalized. Clients with that quality are more able to receive support and develop trust. When that happens, letting go of EMPs is easier. Even with significant EMPs, the stakes are lower and change is easier when a deeply held bias says things will work out for the best.

What cognitive scientists like Kahneman were most interested in were common examples of irrationality, such as loss aversion, a tendency to focus on avoiding losses when it would be more successful to pursue gains. This is a simple example of the inner mind influencing conscious decision-making. It is maladaptive and a pattern, but not entrenched, which is why people are more likely to read Kahneman than to seek psychotherapy to overcome problems with their investment strategies.

To summarize how the EMP phenomenon relates to cognitive science, when the inner self has become detached from the rest of the mind, System 1 and System 2 are more clearly and cleanly separate and distinct. In contrast, in relatively healthy functioning, the two minds operate in partnership, and the distinctions are blurred. Thus, the times when it is most accurate to think of the inner mind as distinct are those when the solution to a problem has become isolated and fixed, which is fundamentally characteristic of EMPs and the territory of psychotherapy.

This isolation of parts of our functioning has long been observed by clinicians. Consistent with this view, the healing process in psychotherapy has sometimes been described as the *integration* of parts of the mind that have been at odds.

INNER SELVES AS THE AGENTS BEHIND EMPS

So far, we've built a picture of inner selves as purposeful agents valiantly fighting for our survival. They do this, based on understandable but outdated notions of the nature of the threat and the best strategy for our protection.

These inner selves often think and act much like children or even mammalian pets. Their information processing is based on information held in nonverbal form and uses associative or metaphorical logic to make if-then decisions comparing and contrasting new information with past experience. The apparatus that supports their calculations has been shaped by evolution, with many preset features as well as biological adjustments that influence results. Remarkably, they are endowed with the ability to form plans and the motivational systems to see them implemented and taken to completion.

Portrait of Inner Selves: Robert

This is a true story, which I have the privilege of recounting because the client, the late Robert Oxnam, wrote about his dissociative identity disorder in his book, *A Fractured Mind* (2005). It was a Saturday in the early 1990s. My beeper went off, and when I returned the call, Robert, in a voice that was clearly shaken, told me that he had nearly been caught shoplifting at his marine hardware store. This might not have been so remarkable in a psychiatric practice, but he was three years my senior and president of the prestigious Asia Society in New York. Soon after, he was in my office, and suddenly his voice changed. A distinctly different Robert appeared, one who didn't know me but eventually started to talk. He was mistrustful at first but soon began to connect as he told me what had happened. The conversation went on for most of the hour. Then, over a few seconds, he faded away, and the original Robert reappeared. I had the strange experience of telling the version of him I knew well that he was sharing his body with another self, who had, indeed, intended to shoplift.

This was not my first encounter with dissociated identities. In Robert's case, the change of voice, manner, and behavior was impossible to miss. From that session on, a new phase of treatment began. Before long, Robert produced a map of the metaphorical castle where his many selves lived. Each one had split off under specific crisis conditions and had remained distinct and frozen in time. During the treatment, they began to grow and evolve until they developed relationships with one another. As they came to appreciate and empathize with one another, they slowly grew into a functioning unit. At the end of our work, Robert was much like the rest of us, one person with a few different sides to himself, suited to different situations. The main difference was that the variations were more distinct and dramatic than for most of us, but information was now shared freely between them and when he produced art, they were functioning as one whole. Robert went on to give hope and encouragement to many others struggling with dissociative identity disorder.

From experiences like the one with Robert, it became a familiar part of my work life to have three-way conversations, speaking to one self, while knowing another was listening. The experience taught me a lot about how children experience danger and turmoil and how they find ways to cope. My work with dissociation led me to realize how much the inner authors of EMPs operate in ways not so different from Robert's inner selves.

FIVE WAYS THE INNER MIND EXERTS ITS INFLUENCE

In Chapter 2, EMPs are defined as including not only products of the inner mind's information processing but also the outward adaptations we identify as patterns of response. Now, let's look in detail at how the inner mind produces those embodied responses. There are five pathways, each of which is important for psychotherapy.

1. **Activating voluntary movements:** The inner mind has direct connections to voluntary muscles and can trigger an automatic vocalization or movement, for example, letting out an exclamation or jumping back from a horrifying sight.
2. **Bodily regulation:** The inner mind has extensive control over body regulation. Some is done through the autonomic nervous system, controlling functions like heart rate and breathing. Since the brain is part of the body, it can even regulate aspects of itself, like the growth of neurons and connections. The brain can also regulate its own workings, such as in paying attention. Hormones are controlled through the hypothalamic-pituitary-adrenal (HPA) axis, affecting multiple body systems, especially those focused on readiness to deal with stress. Even gene expression and transmission can be affected through epigenetics.

   However, the direct bodily effects most relevant to psychotherapy are *affects*, the result of the brain controlling bodily functions like tears, facial expressions, and the hairs on the arms. Both clients and therapists make extensive use of the fact that these bodily responses are not voluntary. Since they bypass consciousness, they register as providing authentic information about the inner mind. They can help clients trust the therapist and help the therapist read what is happening in the client's inner mind, not to mention their value as indicators of what is going on in ourselves.

In psychotherapy, short-term bodily responses like affects are the most relevant to the techniques we use. Many techniques from different orientations and therapies have the effect of activating nonconscious emotions as well as creating a communication channel between the inner self and consciousness. Affect is our main indicator of success in this. The other, more long-term effects listed above, while important, are not emphasized here because they have not had much influence on the design and techniques of psychotherapies. They are not as relevant to psychotherapy technique because they are not direct targets of our efforts. In the end, psychotherapy and the framework developed here are narrowly focused on helping clients develop new, healthier patterns of adaptation and on the information processing that determines the need for EMPs and selection of threat responses. Within the critical area of changing the way the inner mind processes information, the presence of affect is our main way of knowing the process has begun and how it works.

Next, we turn to three *indirect* routes by which the inner mind exerts its influence on our conscious lives. These are the ways the inner mind influences conscious experience and decision-making.

3. **Automatic thoughts:** This and the next two routes are vitally important in understanding how the inner mind influences conscious decision-making. Returning to the concept of an evolutionarily determined competition between the nonconscious inner mind and the conscious one, the inner mind is set up to project information into consciousness much as a computer projects data onto a screen to inform decisions by a human operator. Automatic thoughts are an important part of the overall information the inner mind projects into consciousness.

   Dramatic examples are rationalizations arising in consciousness, often artfully crafted to influence decision-making. Take, for example, the situation of trying to lose weight by dieting. When we manage to resist the impulses to eat, the inner mind has many tricks left. It resorts to obsessive thoughts, rationalizations, and momentary impulses. It is also able to disguise its goals using the principle of one thing leading to another. This means tempting us to take minor steps, with us not realizing that they will inevitably lead to a result we don't consciously want.
4. **Conscious feelings:** The nonconscious emotions of the inner mind act as precursors leading to the construction of conscious feelings.

Those feelings then have important influences on our decisions. Anger, fear, grief, anticipation of pleasure or pain, for example, or less obviously, feelings of uneasiness, something missing, or something needed, are powerfully influential. When their influence is resisted, they tend to grow stronger. Clinical observation often points to instances when such feelings are purposeful in influencing decisions toward goals determined by the inner mind and its EMPs.

5. **Conscious impulses:** The inner mind can also trigger conscious impulses, thoughts that push us to do something immediately. Impulses are frequently the vehicle for overriding or simply bypassing conscious will and wisdom. They often lead to behaviors consistent with the goals of an EMP. It is also important to include impulses *not* to take an action. Procrastination, for example, is usually manifested by an impulse not to perform an action that might otherwise be contemplated. Of particular importance, impulses toward not doing are one of the main tools of EMPs that lead to developmental arrest.

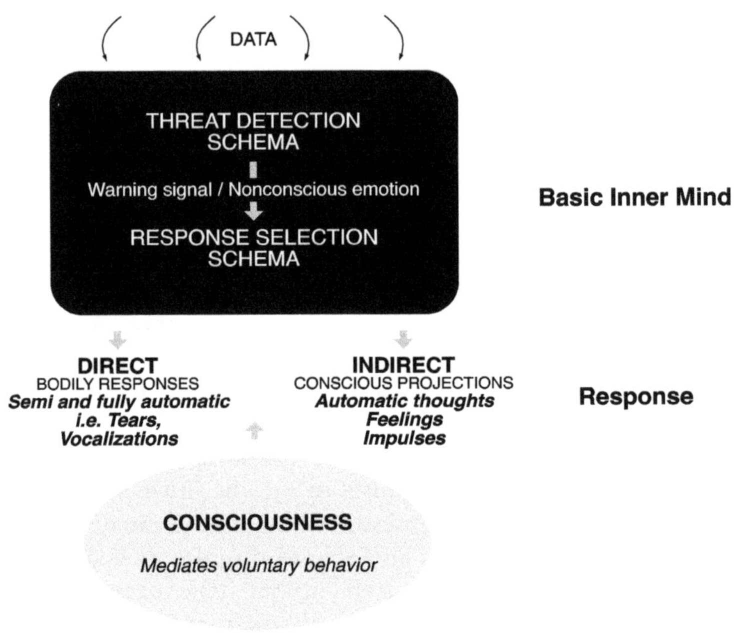

Figure 4.1 Two Direct Products; Three Indirect Via Consciousness

The Inner Mind's Role in Our Lives

These five pathways are the conduits for a large part of what it is to be human. As advertisers and politicians know, they provide the greatest part of our passion and much of our decision-making. That's why advertisers and marketers who want to influence our choices favor nonverbal cues, connotation, imagery, and metaphor. If they didn't want to influence our inner mind, then their communications would be more like scientific journal articles, appealing purely to intellect and formal logic, while avoiding rhetoric and imagery targeting the inner mind.

Between direct influences and those that are mediated by consciousness and voluntary control, inner selves have a significant power to shape our outward decisions and behavior. While inner selves are the originators of the content and drive behind EMPs, there are also many ways the inner mind's influence is healthy and positive, providing an essential counterbalance to conscious will and formal logic. Given the power and influence of inner minds, understanding how and why they work could be one of the most important areas of knowledge to acquire, not just for doing therapy, but for practically every other part of life.

In the next chapter, we'll look more closely at what happens in the therapy room. We'll examine how four selves, two conscious and two inner ones, interact as we develop and follow a plan to help our client to a more satisfactory life.

Key Points

- The "inner mind" is an informal term for the autonomous, nonconscious, subcortical, survival-oriented brain that is closely analogous to similar structures in other mammals.
- When the inner mind's survival circuits form EMPs, they become frozen in time. As such, the EMPs function like inner selves, with goals, strategies, motivation, and even the ability to monitor progress over a lifetime.
- The concept of inner selves provides a description that is more complete than the concepts of transference or cognitive distortion, which are among the products of inner selves.
- Personification of the authors of EMPs can be useful in hypothesizing about their origin and can even be helpful in clinical work.
- Evolutionary biology supports the idea that the inner self is older and more basic, while consciousness is a more recent addition.

- Whether animals experience emotion can be debated, but there is evidence that nonconscious precursors to emotion have powerful effects on animal and human behavior.
- Cognitive science recognizes the concepts of thinking fast and thinking slow, where the first one is characteristic of the inner mind and operates autonomously.
- The inner mind has direct control over bodily functions and regulation, including tears, tone of voice, breathing, hormones, etc.
- The inner mind has the indirect ability to influence voluntary choices using automatic thoughts, feelings, and impulses to do and not to do.
- Addiction and obesity are two examples that show the depth and power of the inner mind to influence behavior against conscious intentions.

REFERENCES

Da Silva, S. (2023). System 1 vs. system 2 thinking. *Psych*, *5*(1), 1–10.

Evans, J. (2003). In two minds: Dual-process accounts of reasoning. *Trends in Cognitive Sciences*, 7, 454–459.

Kahneman, D. (2011). *Thinking, fast and slow*. Farrar, Straus and Giroux.

Oxnam, R. B. (2005). *A fractured mind: My life with multiple personality disorder*. Hyperion.

Panksepp, J., & Biven, L. (2012). *The archaeology of mind: Neuroevolutionary origins of human emotions* (Norton series on interpersonal neurobiology). W. W. Norton & Company.

Schwartz, R. (2013). Moving from acceptance toward transformation with Internal Family Systems Therapy (IFS). *Journal of Clinical Psychology*, *69*(8), 805–816.

Smith, R., & Lane, R. (2016). Unconscious emotion: A cognitive neuroscientific perspective. *Neuroscience & Biobehavioral Reviews*, *69*, 216–238.

Whelton, W. (2004). Emotional processes in psychotherapy: Evidence across therapeutic modalities. *Clinical Psychology & Psychotherapy*, *11*, 58–71.

CHAPTER 5
The Plan

In this chapter, we'll use what we know so far and apply it to the operation of helping clients trade outdated EMPs for more satisfactory ways of responding. In the process, we'll look at the interaction between four selves: the conscious client, the client's inner self, and similar parts of the therapist.

One of the significant differences between the cognitive-behavioral (CBT) orientation and the psychodynamic orientation is that behavioral therapies focus on problem-solving. They focus on eliminating symptoms and problem behaviors. Meanwhile, the psychodynamic orientation is ambivalent about whether it is a process that results in symptom relief of a problem-solving procedure.

To clarify this issue, let's go back in history. Freud began as a trauma therapist, describing cases where hysterical conversion symptoms like Anna O's were caused by trauma (Freud & Breuer, 1895/1955). As previously dissociated experiences came to consciousness with affect, symptoms disappeared. Making the unconscious conscious seemed to be all it took. There was no need for a plan other than allowing the patient to speak freely then seeing relief of symptoms take place, simply through being heard. As a Victorian scientist, Freud saw himself as a neutral, objective observer. He downplayed the role of the therapist or the relationship, except to see it as a blank canvas on which the inner mind's concerns were painted.

As psychoanalysis evolved, it moved more toward a process as opposed to a plan for symptom resolution. The unconscious would impose its conflicts and wishes on the canvas of the transference, that is, relationships from the past were projected onto the therapist, and the resolution of those conflicts would steer the course of the analysis.

DOI: 10.4324/9781003619659-6

Glen Gabbard, writer of a classic textbook of psychodynamic therapy (Gabbard, 2017) suggests that psychodynamically oriented psychotherapy follows both a plan and a process. An initial evaluation takes note of problem patterns, but the unfolding of the therapy follows something more like the Freudian process than a problem-solving plan.

With an understanding of the infrastructure, we will see how it is natural to do both. Understanding the processes, we will be able to guide them according to a plan, but one that evolves as we work. It will leave room for discovery along the way but will be structured around the ultimate goal of helping clients trade EMPs for more satisfactory responses to the same inputs and circumstances. Let's turn, then, to how we can accomplish this.

FOUR SELVES IN THE ROOM

The client comes to therapy with a primary pain point or complaint, which we relate to one or more EMPs. We recognize that the authors of the EMPs are inner selves with their own goals and agendas based on outdated attempts to solve major life challenges. In this way, there are two persons in the room on the client side. We work actively with the fact that the goals of the adult and inner selves may or may not coincide.

For now, while recognizing that we, as therapists, ourselves, have both a conscious mind and an inner mind, we'll treat them as one, in the expectation that they will be working in partnership. In that way, we can think of ourselves primarily as a third person in the room. Inevitably, though, there will be instances of countertransference, when the therapist's inner self becomes split from the mainstream and imposes its own agenda on the therapeutic situation. At those times, there will be four people actively in the room. For now, we'll leave out influences from beyond the consulting room such as family dynamics, though they are critically important and will be discussed in Chapter 11.

Seeking accurate empathy is a process, but focusing that effort on an identified EMP makes it into a plan. Bringing the psychodynamic and behavioral orientations under one roof, it is natural to have both a problem-solving plan and to recognize a process in which EMPs and their inner authors' agendas first reveal themselves, then become the focus of plans to help the client trade outdated solutions for more satisfactory ones. Since we may not be able to see all of the EMP layers at the outset, this is an unfolding process, but ultimately, we are looking at therapy as a way of solving problems to improve life. Going forward in this chapter, we look at how such multifaceted plans play out in actual practice.

An Adult Client Comes for Help

Maria, a 36-year-old marketing executive, enters psychotherapy after experiencing increasing anxiety at work. She describes feeling overwhelmed, with difficulty concentrating and a growing fear that she will lose control in a professional setting. Maria also reports chronic difficulties in romantic relationships, often ending them abruptly when she feels criticized or rejected.

Maria was born to immigrant parents and was the youngest of four children. Her father was emotionally distant and frequently traveled for work, while her mother struggled with depression. Maria often felt overlooked and learned to be self-reliant from a young age. She recalled being praised for her achievements but rarely comforted when upset.

Maria became a high achiever in school, driven by a desire for approval. She described her teenage years as lonely, with few close friends. In college, she excelled academically but struggled with intense self-criticism and perfectionism. Romantic relationships were short-lived and tumultuous, marked by fears of abandonment and emotional volatility.

In the initial evaluation, Maria's anxiety over loss of control at work was identified as the top-level EMP, designed by her inner mind to function both as a cry for help and a way to avoid some even worse loss of control. The focus then moved quickly to the second layer, an EMP leading her to seek some form of relief by screaming out loud and causing trouble at work. She had no idea why any part of her mind should be upset, since she was successful at work and doing well in her adult life, except that she hadn't met the right man. Let's picture her therapy process.

THE WORK

The definition of work is applying force to an object and moving it over a distance against resistance, in other words, going from point A to point B against ®, resistance, arising from a nonconscious fear of change.

A-----------®-----------B

When we begin to feel a client's resistance to change, it means we are finally engaged in doing the work of therapy. Until then, we are in an exploratory mode, seeking to understand the architecture of the client's problems so we can begin to envision a pathway to change. As we start on that pathway, we begin to sense that progress won't be so easy. In working with Maria, the first step of therapy is encouraging her to become aware that her inner self is not as happy as she imagines.

Her insistence that everything had been fine indicates that her inner mind was braced and ready to put up some resistance to any attempt to get close to the source of the violent inner energy she perceived as terribly dangerous. At the same time, her inner self yearned to be heard. Between the two, the desire to share with an empathic witness wins out step-by-step, and she begins to reveal more.

Adult Maria is invited to explore her inner mind. She gradually begins to recall childhood memories of feeling invisible and experiencing pressure to be the perfect daughter. The EMP that is causing her inner mind to experience pressure to scream out loud begins to make sense as the consequence of a childhood prohibition against complaining. She was supposed to be the perfect child who never complained and gladly sacrificed the childhood carefreeness her emotional development needed. The work is beginning to focus on her self-prohibition and its entrenchment. As her fear of revealing her early life unhappiness softens, a new inner fear and resistance appear.

We begin to experience stronger entrenchment as accurate empathy gives a fuller understanding of the facts of her early life. Empathy for herself begins to bring emotion to the surface. Her discomfort increases as she faces the more central work of experiencing and processing the residual pain of what was an insoluble problem when she was young. The new, adult solution, which can replace her EMP's work-focused anxiety, will be to dare to share her emotions with her therapist, which will lead naturally to acceptance and making peace with her painful early life. She will also learn in a more general way to share her troubles with appropriate others, rather than presenting a perfect front, as she had learned to do in childhood. Later, she will try this new skill out in other places in her life, overcoming her outdated fear of being "real." She will learn that her old ability to hide her distress may still be valuable at work, but not in her private life. She may also find that her failure to find the right man came from her own failure to reveal enough of herself to bond with anyone.

Taking entrenchment into account, we can further expand our definition of what psychotherapy does. The goal of psychotherapy can be expanded further to this:

Helping clients, against the resistance presented by entrenchment, trade their mind's less-than-optimal adaptations for more satisfactory ones by updating the inner mind's information processing to generate a different and more satisfactory response to the same or similar conditions.

This view of the plan is compatible with both the psychodynamic orientation and a behavioral one. For psychodynamic therapists, we look at the unconscious mind as the inner mind fulfilling its evolution-based protective role. For the behavioral orientation, despite a tradition of avoiding speculation about the nonconscious mind, I am suggesting that it is clinically responsible and valuable to see the subcortical mind as an active agent, evolved to solve problems utilizing core beliefs and automatic thoughts for purposes of survival. While our understanding of what goes on in a given inner mind is provisional, it is nevertheless highly useful when seeking enduring change to outdated patterns of response. As accurate empathy brings emotionally engaged clarity, the client learns new skills for coping with strong emotions.

MODELS OF TREATMENT

Looking at the plan, we also need to compare this approach to other methods currently in use to treat emotional troubles. For example, today, people with similar issues to Maria's are being treated under the medical model in which the patient (not client) is a victim of illness and a passive recipient of treatment. In contrast, the "rehab model" used here sees the problem as an outdated solution and the *client* is an active participant in shifting to a more satisfactory solution.

The Medical Model

Today, much of Western medicine follows the medical model in which the patient *has* a disorder (Barber, 2012). That model talks about patients, not clients. It works like the treatment for pneumonia or arthritis in the knee. The patient's job is to describe symptoms to help the doctor follow a preset decision tree. The doctor has a road map and applies the correct label to place the patient in a category, which determines the treatment. The patient then becomes the passive recipient of treatment and, hopefully, gets better.

The medical model has become so deeply accepted in the US and world culture that clients often announce, "I have depression." They label themselves, expecting that that information will help the doctor know what treatment to prescribe. They imagine walking out with a prescription, and everything will be fine. The model is popular because it minimizes professional time, avoids the patient having to face painful emotions, and is favorable to corporate interests in that it perpetuates the myth that just finding the right protocol will be enough to cure the "illness." The only downside is that, unless the problem is mainly of biological origin, it doesn't work well over time.

It's not that there aren't psychological and emotional problems primarily of biological origin (See Appendix). In these cases, biological treatments may be helpful. In such cases, there may also be psychological adaptations to biological problems that can be improved with psychotherapy. It is no less common to have situations where biological and psychological factors are mixed. In Maria's case, for example, she may have had a predilection for anxiety, but the main cause of her troubles was psychological, and so was the most appropriate treatment.

If the medical model were applied in Maria's case, an antidepressant would most likely have been prescribed, with the effect of suppressing emotions in general. Her anxiety might have been diminished, while her ability to contain her unhappiness and maintain her façade could be maintained, at least for a while. Underneath, her troubles would not have changed, and her inability to form a relationship would remain in place. In my opinion, this treatment would not be appropriate, even though she may have had a genetic predilection for excessive anxiety.

A consequence of excessive use of the medical model can be treating the diagnosis instead of the person. In a more serious example, Fiona, a college student, became genuinely and seriously depressed. The doctor gave antidepressants, which did not work because the depression was a symptom, not an isolated illness. The cause of her depressed feelings was a lifelong pattern of seeking love by performing, which never worked, and left her in increasing despair. Seeing that the treatment was failing, the doctor recommended shock therapy, which also failed to address the problem. That triggered a further escalation of hopelessness.

Following a second opinion, the plan was changed to helping Fiona let go of her reliance on performance and to adopt the scary new practice of persisting in presenting her genuine, vulnerable self in relationships at college. In the end, a lot of warmth and encouragement from a team of helpers allowed this warm-hearted and appealing young person to discover that, in place of the EMP that tried to use performance, her human qualities began to win the love she needed. Her depression lifted, and she was eventually able to discontinue the medications. This was a somewhat unusual case in that her strength was her ability to accept the warmth she so desired. She had a degree of "basic trust." That is not always the case. The best alternatives to replace EMPs are often pre-existing strengths and skills.

The Recovery Model

As in the cases of Maria and the ultimately successful treatment of the college student, a more realistic model for psychotherapy is the "recovery model" (Barber, 2012). There, it is assumed that, whatever the diagnosis, the client can gain improvement in functioning and life satisfaction. It is assumed that the problem is an inner misunderstanding of how best to live life, and that the treatment will help the individual access previously unavailable options. The therapy will help trade old, maladaptive patterns for new, more satisfactory ones. The work will consist of coming to understand the nature and triggers of maladaptive responses, using positive relationships to help overcome fears of change, and to make use of existing strengths and new patterns to replace outdated EMPs. In this model, the client is anything but passive, and the therapist is a facilitator, helping to harness change processes that are already native to humankind.

Returning to Maria's experience, the psychodynamic approach might be to listen empathically to her intellectual discussion of her role as the perfect child and to wait as she discovers more passionate feelings underneath. Interpretation might be used to clarify that her intellectualizing and perfectionism are serving an outdated purpose.

A CBT approach emphasizes skill building. It would be to teach her that her anxiety doesn't come from any real danger and that there are techniques like breathing and mindfulness to make it possible to tolerate anxiety, realizing that it is a product of her inner mind and does not require a response.

What the present framework might suggest would be a combination of both, a more active stance in helping her champion her inner self and its desire to be heard. Informed by the idea of a separate inner self, the therapy would encourage her to learn that expressing feelings with affect is not only acceptable, but far healthier. It would also represent a way to bypass the need for screaming out loud. She would be encouraged to compare her outdated inner rule never to express strong emotions with a new rule that sharing emotions with an empathic witness is a positive and healthy thing to do. Furthermore, she might be encouraged to accept that she was never a perfect child, only a real and vibrant young human.

By that time, it will be apparent that the failure of finding the right man arose from another layer of EMP in which she was choosing ungiving men, much like her parents, and hoping unrealistically that being perfect would make them into warm and giving partners.

HOW TO BUILD A PLAN

Now that we have some understanding of how different models work, let's get back to our plan to trade outdated EMPs for more satisfactory ways of responding. We start out with a rational adult client like Maria, the first participant in the room. She is requesting help, but how do we get from there to a plan? Here are the steps that will lead to the essential components.

- **Step 1. The chief complaint:** We need to listen intently, seeking the most accurate empathy possible regarding just what the client is suffering from. That is critically important for three reasons. First, it is the source of energy and drive to sustain the therapy. Second, accurate empathy about the chief complaint will help build the therapetuic alliance, and third, it will put us on the trail to finding the EMP underneath. So, we inquire in depth, then follow our curiosity by asking for more detail.
- **Step 2. Find the EMP:** This means understanding how the chief complaint is the result of a problem-solving strategy employed by the inner mind. That may not be obvious and may take time to clarify. An EMP may be the direct cause of suffering as in Maria's anxiety, or it may be less direct and more hidden as with her difficulty finding the right man. We still need to find the first layer of EMP to approach before we can embark on a plan.
- **Step 3. Locate the resistance:** The final question that leads to our getting to work is asking ourselves and possibly the client, why the needed change has not already happened. That is where the entrenchment or resistance to positive change resides.
- **Step 4. Begin the work:** Finally, we begin to focus on how to help our client overcome their involuntary, inner resistance to make the needed changes. We do need to be thoughtful here, as this resistance is not just being obstinate; it is probably a younger self, trying to do the right things to avoid a disaster. And let's not forget the possibility that her reluctance is that she does not yet trust the therapy. Imagine inner Maria letting go. She's rightfully afraid that would mean screaming out loud at work and losing her job. Why would she want to do that? She'll need to find sources of confidence and courage, as well as learning to use the therapy as an appropriate channel for her intense emotions.

From here on, we discuss how to approach the work itself. But before we can do that, we need clarity about who we are working with.

Inner Selves Are Participants, Too

You may recognize that Maria's inner self entering the therapy room is an example of what psychodynamic therapy would call transference.

Maria's initially intellectualized description of her early self as a perfect child was designed to satisfy a therapist she imagined would expect nothing but an idealized version of the truth. In her mind, the therapist will be unwilling to hear negative emotions. Psychodynamic therapy would correctly describe this as a distortion in her perception of the therapist, based on her past. There is more to it.

I sometimes use the word transference still, but my understanding of it has changed dramatically. What made the difference was recognizing the role of inner selves in the problems psychotherapy is designed to treat. The transformation in my own thinking began with a series of blog posts that became a resource for clients experiencing intense attachment to their therapist. They described feeling that they couldn't survive without the person of their therapist. Seeking to understand the phenomenon, it was clear that powerful inner selves were trying, by any means possible, to solve problems of early deprivation by getting what they had missed from a kind and caring therapist.

As stories accumulated in comments to the blog, I documented their struggles in an e-book, *Attachment to Your Therapist: A Conversation* (2016). The experience led me to a much more personified view of transference. That was the beginning. I was shocked at the number of therapeutic disasters they recounted, which convinced me to change my professional focus to looking for ways to help therapists build greater skill and confidence in handling the intensity of relationships with inner selves.

What became clear to me was that, as described in Chapter 4, while transference is accurate in capturing the perceptual distortions, descriptions often fail to recognize the drive and purposefulness behind the phenomenon. A more complete and accurate view of what I was witnessing in my own practice and through the blog posts was a powerful and determined inner self with a plan invented long ago, based on views and strategies frozen in time. Furthermore, it had specific goals and an life-saving drive to put them into effect.

THREE SELVES IN THE ROOM

We have built up a picture of the adult client and a spectrum of inner selves bringing their influence into the room. Now, let's look at how we therapists handle the reality of having two clients at the same time in the same room. For now, we'll think of the therapist functioning as one person, an effective partnership between a subcortical inner mind and a conscious rational self, where both are working together to facilitate the client's progress. In other words, we now have three selves in the room.

Introducing the Inner Self to the Adult Client

It often falls to the therapist to introduce the idea that an inner self with an independent agenda is causing problems. The first response of most clients is usually quite negative. "How can I get rid of that pesky inner self?" The reason is that early in life, most of us internalize values favoring being "grown-up" and in control of ourselves. Those values motivate us to act in a rational and mature way, but they also set us up to be judgmental and intolerant of our wayward inner selves.

Our first job as therapists is to help the adult client come to accept that the best way to help children grow is through encouragement and empathy. Too many clients have experienced judgment and punishment from role models. It may feel strange for an adult client to think of befriending a young part, but that is what works best. Here, again, the traditional response to transference is to interpret, in a neutral way, the client's distorted perceptions. That does little to promote a positive attitude toward the author of those perceptions. Hopefully, an experienced therapist will intuitively understand the need for a warmer approach, but when we adopt a personified view of the inner self, it becomes crystal clear that we need to form a relationship with both client selves. Without an empathic connection with the inner self, we will have a hard time being effective in helping this stuck inner person rejoin the mainstream of the client's life.

Partnering with the Adult to Help the Inner Self

What should begin to be apparent is that our adult client can and should become an ally in helping the inner self outgrow their maladaptive patterns. That changes the dynamics and the relationships. The adult client is no longer a passive witness to our work with the inner self but has gained an equal or greater role. As the adult is able to overcome their shame about having a stowaway inside, they will hopefully embrace their role as a healer.

How can we talk to our two clients at the same time? It is very much like a family conversation where we are addressing one member in terms appropriate for their age and development, while being aware of the others present. Internal family systems therapy says we should address younger selves directly. That works naturally for some clients and not for others. We might switch back and forth or use simpler language to make sure a younger participant is not left out. "We both know that your young self was badly hurt and is afraid of trusting. We'll both (therapist and adult client) need to be gentle and very reliable to help her know we understand her fragility." To the inner self: "I'm aware that a young part is there, and I'm speaking to that part to let you know I understand." And I'm being especially sure not to make or imply promises I am not sure I can keep.

The keys are tact, consistency, and respect. We want to demonstrate in our attitude an awareness of caring for all participants. That is a natural outcome of accurate empathy combined with the dual goals of helping the adult adopt a stance of acceptance while helping the inner self experience understanding, caring, and encouragement in taking the risks of trying new ways to respond.

INNER CRITICS, THE SOURCES OF SHAME AND GUILT

So far, I haven't mentioned an important type of inner self, the inner critic. I have not focused on it because the EMPs they participate in are quite different from other EMPs. This section is brief, but of very great importance, so please read carefully. This kind of inner self will take up disproportionately large amounts of therapy time and effort.

Humans are different from our mammalian ancestors in having an active self-policing function utilizing shame and guilt as deterrents and pride as a reinforcer to keep us in line with social expectations and out of trouble. It's called the conscience. Given the primacy of social cohesion for human survival, it is not surprising that this system has evolved with an architecture different from other mammalian survival circuits. Specifically, it involves judging our own behavior according to internalized standards. Those standards include values, as well as attitudes, ideals, and prohibitions. The judgment takes place mainly in the cortex, but feelings of shame and guilt appear to be products of the same powerful subcortical survival circuits as other dreaded inner experiences—thus constituting the "enforcement arm" of a complete self-policing system. As long as the values are healthy, then the system is positive and beneficial, but, too often, EMPs arise from internalizing faulty values and attitudes designed to save the self from some terrible consequence.

These powerful influences, while originating in the cortex, appear to make use of subcortical circuits originally designed for mammalian submissive behavior. Thus, shame induces experiences of feeling mortified and wanting to shrink to nothing and disappear as the emotional part of the experience. Not surprisingly, the internalized standards that lie at the core of the system are particularly resistant to change. If they weren't, then temptation would always win. The inner selves that administer this system are our inner critics. The unhealthy internal standards they embrace appear to be subject to the same change mechanisms as other implicit learnings, but inner critics are decidedly more resistant to any attempt to soften those standards. The entrenchment here is guarding internal values against what is perceived as corruption and impropriety.

In clinical practice it often happens that the original fear of being hurt can be resolved in therapy, but lingering waves of shame show that this conscience-based self-critical function is still intact. The system is working as designed, but we'll have to make changes to unhealthy internal standards.

The Conscience Is also Subject to Pathology

Whenever we see inappropriate shame or guilt, it's fair to assume that an inner critic is at work. More importantly, the inner critic is only doing its job. The real culprit is the unhealthy internalized standard being used to judge the self. That is what needs to change. The most common examples are coping with harshness or abuse by identifying with the aggressor. Taking the side of the abuser may function to keep some kind of connection and ward off the utter aloneness of being rejeccted or devalued. That means internalizing the abuser's negative attitude toward the self. The inner self may also be able to turn passive into active by getting there first in attacking the self. Children sometimes invent their own values as deterrents to help them control behaviors likely to get them in trouble. These are the "internal electric fences" mentioned earlier. For example, as in the case of John in Chapter 3, being attacked repeatedly for being "weak" can lead to internalizing a value system against any form of dependency or weakness. From then on, John's main dread is not being hurt but experiencing self-induced shame as a result of needy behavior or even thoughts.

Anorexia nervosa is an interesting example of such an internal electric fence. A strong value system promotes control over food. When the client eats, he or she feels tremendous shame and disgust. The underlying dynamic is that control over food has become a proxy for control over emotional neediness and a symbolic victory over experiences of emotional deprivation. This formulation is supported in the literature by Munro et al. (2017).

In therapy, challenging such an inner critic is especially difficult. Pathological values are usually rationalized as healthy and necessary. Very often, the adult client comes to the defense of the inner critic. We generally assume that Jiminy Cricket, the personification of our conscience, is always right. The idea of values being wrong seems alien and suspect. Clients will insist, "Yes, I am worthless, look at how little I have accomplished in life." When we question their values, they may turn against us, accusing the therapist of being immoral or corrupt. For this reason, we need to be very careful about challenging internalized values, attitudes, ideals, and prohibitions. The job still needs to be done, but we need to acknowledge the intense resistance associated with unhealthy shame and self-criticism.

The first step in supporting change is developing intellectual clarity about the traumatic source of an unhealthy value system and clarity that it is maladaptive and should change. The next step is what I call "civil disobedience," that is, adopting a voluntary behavior change, acting against an internalized but pathological standard. While encouraging this value-challenging behavior, it is also important to warn the client to expect it to lead to a backlash of intense shame or guilt. The appropriate response is to persist anyway, showing the inner self that healthy behavior is actually safe. The temptation to compromise with the inner critic should be resisted, as it tends to reinforce the unhealthy values instead of challenging them. Halfway measures are a bit like negotiating a compromise with terrorists. They tend to reinforce the old values rather than favoring change.

The Spiral-Bound Book

Especially in practicing civil disobedience, it is too easy for clients to lose track of how their inner self is working to justify the status quo and how they need to stay focused on change. Without realizing it, they often slip back into old patterns of self-judgment. In this and any other situation where we are hoping to show the inner self a better way, it is too easy for clients to lose both empathy and clarity about needed voluntary changes. What I sometimes suggest is a spiral-bound book that lies open on two pages at once. On the left, clients put themselves in the shoes of their inner self and write down how it sees the situation and its ideas of how to solve it. On the right, I ask them to represent the healthy adult point of view. Following this practice helps the client develop accurate empathy for their own inner self as well as clarity about how and why the inner self's strategy is ripe for replacement with a better set of values, attitudes, ideals, or prohibitions.

Dealing With Deprived Inner Selves' Wishes and Needs

The discussion of how inner selves deal with deprivation raises the question of how to handle inner selves' plans for us to fill in areas of deprivation. Not infrequently, inner selves adopt the strategy of waiting for some nice person to come and fill in what was missing. The strategy is that they will be spared having to face the painful hopelessness of realizing that their childhood needs will never be met. And of course, the therapist steps right into the role of supplying the missing understanding, love, support, or attention. Here is an example of how this can play out.

Thomas, a highly intelligent 46-year-old professional, is in therapy with an analytically oriented therapist. He attends sessions faithfully, says what is on his mind, and eventually dares to tell his therapist that he would appreciate some practical tips on life skills. His request is curiously out of sync with the age and accomplishments of the adult client, but the therapist fails to notice and answers, "This is psychoanalytically oriented therapy, and advice giving is not part of what we do." The client, deeply disappointed, doesn't argue and keeps going to therapy, but his inner self loses hope. The energy drains from the therapy. Eventually, he decides he has gotten as much benefit as he can and drops out of treatment.

What happened? Do you remember from Chapter 1, the therapy consultant's dictum? *When there is a problem in therapy, it's right in front of you and has to do with the relationship.* Thomas was diligently following his therapist's instructions to say what came to mind, but as expected in psychodynamic therapy, transference happened. A child-client awoke. As a child, he had been severely deprived of fathering. In a very young way, his inner self had devised a plan. The child's solution was to avoid the pain by waiting, keeping hope alive, and eventually finding a substitute to reverse the deprivation. We can imagine that, for a small child, accepting his dad's inadequacy was far beyond his capacity. Instead, he would wait as long as necessary to find a nice, trustworthy older man to fill in what he had not received from his father. That way, he would never have to go through painful acceptance and the process of grieving for what he had missed.

Instead of talking tactfully about his client's childlike wish, the therapist invoked the rules and re-created precisely the same hurtful disappointment this young self had experienced early in life. That's a good segue into talking about the fourth person in the room.

THE FOURTH PERSON IN THE ROOM

The therapist's response to Thomas didn't come from a well-trained and experienced adult self. It came from the therapist's inner self, triggered by the client's request. Perhaps his subcortical inner mind was set in motion by the demand that he break the rules and give advice. Perhaps the therapist had experienced mortifying shame the day his supervisor admonished him not to gratify his client's wishes. Whatever the specifics, we are witnessing a full-blown countertransference, which, unfortunately, was not recognized and went on to cause the serious consequence of a failed therapy.

Had this rupture been recognized, the therapist would have had a chance to repair it. Repair first involves acknowledging one's own contribution to the break, if any. Next, we seek accurate empathy to understand the impact on the client. That and an apology from the therapist is often enough to repair the rift. If we have worked hard to maintain a good relationship, clients want to forgive. Furthermore, in Thomas's case, exploration would have revealed the central issue in his therapy, a deprivation of fathering that left him perpetually waiting and never completing his own maturation into emotional adulthood.

Picking Up the Pieces

A few months later, I had the privilege of cleaning up the damage when Thomas appeared in my office and spoke about his previous attempt at therapy. I did what I often do in cases like this, where the client is far from being ready to look warmly and objectively at his own inner child. I offered to give him whatever tips on life skills I could but suggested at the same time that we would need to seek understanding about the source of his request. What I knew was that the bits of advice I might offer would never fully satisfy his need, and that the yearning would become more clear. Soon, he was able to see that my help, well-meaning as it was, could not give him what his inner self was hoping for. This time, it wasn't a refusal, but doing my genuine best and inevitably falling short, that brought clarity. Finally, it was time for him to go through the very real pain and grief about what he had missed. He needed to do this in the presence of an empathic witness to come to acceptance so that he could move on to become fully adult. That is the work we did. In situatons like this, as with parenting, it is not uncommon that the agent causing the pain is also the empathic witness who helps with healing.

At this point, with a fuller understanding of how and why EMPs are created by inner selves, and how they show up in therapy, let's turn to see how change happens. First, we'll need a thorough understanding of how survival circuits operate. Then we will be able to see how words, nonverbal information, and relationships can bring change to their functioning.

Key Points

- Is psychotherapy a procedure aimed at rapid symptom resolution or a process of transformation addressing the causes of symptoms? As we understand the infrastructure of therapy, we can see better that we don't have to choose.
- The fact that EMPs are layered requires a process of discovery, but in the present model, symptom resolution can be addressed either top-down as envisioned in CBT, or bottom-up utilizing the transformative memory reconsolidation.
- The medical model, popular today, sees the patient as a passive recipient of treatment, which is contrasted with the recovery model presented here in which the client has an active role.
- Steps to building a plan are suggested starting with identification of the relevant EMP, and moving toward fulfilling requirements for transformative change.
- Personification of the inner self is contrasted with the concepts of transference and cognitive distortions, where the inner self brings additional dimensions of purpose, motivation, and persistence over time.
- The subject of talking with inner selves and recruiting the adult self as a partner is like a family conversation with children and adults.
- Inner critics are a special case of EMP, where pathological internalized values, attitudes, ideals, and prohibitions are the basis of EMPs and are particularly resistant to change.
- Needs of inner selves can pose particular problems for therapists and require careful management of expectations.
- The final point is to view countertransference as interference by the therapist's inner self, with its own agendas, to the flow of psychotherapy.

REFERENCES

Barber, M. (2012). Recovery as the new medical model for psychiatry. *Psychiatric services, 63*(3), 277–279.

Freud, S., & Breuer, J. (1895/1955). Studies on Hysteria. In Strachey (Ed.)J. , *The standard edition of the complete psychological works of sigmund freud, Vol. 2*. Random House.

Gabbard, G. O. (2017). *Long-term psychodynamic psychotherapy: A basic text* (3rd ed.). American Psychiatric Publishing.

Munro, C., Randell, L., & Lawrie, S. (2017). An integrative bio-psycho-social theory of Anorexia Nervosa.. *Clinical Psychology & Psychotherapy, 24*(1), 1–21.

Smith, J. (2016). *Attachment to your therapist: A conversation*. Libentia Press.

CHAPTER 6

Inside Every EMP

Now it's time to go inside all EMPs to explain what they are made of and how words, nonverbal information, and relationships can change them.

Recent miracle treatments in medicine have come out of increasingly intimate knowledge of how the body functions. We can take the same approach with psychotherapy. Knowing just how it works will help us track how and where to aim our words and communications. With a fresh level of clarity, it becomes possible to design treatments that wing their way precisely into the places where they can make a difference. That's what we have needed for a long time, but for the first hundred or so years of our profession, the science was not available to show just what makes psychotherapy work.

What Are the Components of EMPs?

For any EMP, we can talk about several different components going into its construction and embodiment as a protective response. Here is a list to get us oriented. Every EMP has the following elements:

- A *threat detection schema*.
- A *warning signal* consisting of a *nonconscious emotion*.
- A *response selection schema* to determine the response.
- Response elements directly affecting the body, including *affects*.
- Automatic *thoughts*, *feelings*, and *impulses* to influence conscious choices.
- *Consequences* of both voluntary and involuntary behaviors.

DOI: 10.4324/9781003619659-7

STEP BY STEP: HOW EMPS WORK

Step 1: Threat Detection

The first stage in the initiation of an EMP is the detection of a threat. The inner mind is constantly monitoring the environment and comparing what it finds with past experiences and expectations to identify and predict possible threats. A threat detection schema is the unit of logic that does that, alternatively described as a *symptom-requiring schema* (Ecker et al., 2024). This bit of procedural memory located in a subcortical structure such as the amygdala, uses predictive coding for pattern recognition to identify threats.

Step 2: Issuing a Warning Signal

When the threat-detecting schema predicts the likelihood of a threat, a warning signal is created through the activation of neurons to communicate the need for a response (Ledoux, 2021). That warning signal, as we have discussed, is in the form of a nonconscious emotion, one of those precursor emotions that go on to activate a second schema that selects the specific response.

Our first indication of this nonconscious action is the appearance of affect, the earliest indication of a response. Going forward, I'll often call the warning signal a *warning signal/nonconscious emotion* to keep both of its faces in view at the same time.

Step 3: Response Selection

A response selection schema—Ecker et al. (2024) call it *solution-defining*—is triggered into action by the warning signal/nonconscious emotion. Response selection works by applying complex rules to determine which response should be used for the specific circumstances. The output triggers a launching of the actual response. Like the threat detection schema, it is stored as procedural memory and uses predictive coding for pattern matching to connect the details of the threat to a specific response.

Responses turn to action via the five pathways described in Chapter 4:

1. Direct, semi-automatic control over musculature (letting out a cry).
2. Direct, automatic control over bodily and brain regulation, including affect.
3. Indirect influence via automatic thoughts.
4. Indirect influence via conscious feelings.
5. Indirect influence via impulses to do (or not to do).

Step 4: Direct Bodily Responses

The first two pathways are the direct ones acting on the body and brain. They are the first to be manifested because they are fast, direct, and are not mediated by conscious "thinking slow." To be complete, in Chapter 4, I catalogued short and long-term bodily responses, pointing out that the short-term ones, particularly bodily affects, are the most relevant to psychotherapy technique. In particular, bodily affects, such as tears or an involuntary facial expression, are our most reliable indicators of proto-emotion coming from the inner mind. They are also indicators that a two-way communication channel has been opened between the inner mind and consciousness. Such a channel will turn out to be vital to therapeutic success.

Step 5: Powerful Influences over Conscious Choice

EMPs use three indirect pathways, automatic thoughts, feelings, and impulses to counterbalance conscious will and to influence decisions. How can we know this? As we look more closely at these, we'll see that they are major determinants of what we think and do. Considering the hypothesis that automatic thoughts, feelings, and impulses are meant to drive us toward the inner mind's plan leads, over time, to a body of favorable clinical evidence. And our inner minds don't let up. They persist and have a great deal of depth and creativity in how they persist until we relent and follow their directives.

Motivation, conscious and nonconscious, is an important component of the inner mind's systems for influencing behavior. We are induced from within to follow up and ensure that the implementation proceeds until it ultimately reaches the inner mind's planned goal. Think about how sensitive we are to closure or the lack of it, or how we naturally focus on the end of a story, expecting a resolution. In both cases, motivation is automatically engaged to encourage us to seek a feeling of completion. In Chapter 11, we will look more closely at motivation.

The power of the inner mind's influence is exemplified in the developed world by the fight against obesity. Recalling the comparison of EMP layers with the defenses of a medieval castle, an inner self has its own layers and depths of strategy for overcoming the conscious reluctance to eat. It may start with hunger pangs, but if they don't work, it begins to project obsessive thoughts into consciousness. Then it follows with impulses. The inner mind is creative. "Maybe I'll just have a small portion." And it knows how to use the trick of one thing leading to another. "I'll just have one," and soon that leads to another and another.

We might also consider a worldwide trend of profiting by offering easy fulfillment of a range of instinctive human needs. Many such products engage the inner mind's power in ways that can promote compulsive use, excess, and damaging consequences. Where profit demands doing everything possible to facilitate consumption, for some individuals this creates an unfair battle. Fighting against their own inner mind's ideas of what is good for survival can manifest as a losing battle.

These examples emphasize the power of the human inner mind to have a major impact on worldwide health, where vast numbers of individuals lives are degraded in ways that are unique to each. Beyond instinctive bodily needs, we can see how EMPs, aiming to protect our social survival, are endemic to human life. Unique individual EMPs are often less obvious but equally costly targets of psychotherapy. They are endowed with the same strong tools and strategies for influencing free will. That is where psychotherapy has a significant role in turning individual tragedies into better lives.

Step 6: Our Modest Capacity to Edit the Expression of EMPs

Despite the power of EMPs, our capacity for thinking slowly utilizing conscious reasoning does give us some ability to recognize actions to avoid, feelings that are not valid, and impulses best not acted upon.

The conscious mind's capacity to edit products of the inner mind opens up the possibility of top-down change, where the client works to manage inputs from the inner mind, substituting different and improved responses. This can, to an extent, lead to better functioning, but the influence of the instinctive inner mind is very strong and tends to find ways to get back to what it considers beneficial. That's why top-down change is often thought of as less enduring.

At the same time, adopting new patterns of response on a top-down basis has a potential benefit that is not always recognized. Conscious efforts to change behavior can create an experiential message that is transmitted to the inner mind, showing that the new behavior is not as dangerous as the inner mind has anticipated. When this takes place in a context where the inner mind's schemas are in an active state, the change mechanism of memory reconsolidation can cause a bottom-up change. In other words, behavioral experience, adopted voluntarily by a client, can function as the very disconfirming information, with which schemas can be rewritten. This will be described further in Chapter 10 on "The Art of Disconfirmation."

Step 7: Consequences of the Embodiments of EMPs

Both directly controlled automatic behaviors and those that result from the inner mind's influences have consequences. Affects have consequences, too. They become inputs into the mind's information processing, where they can trigger responses. Vicious cycles can arise when an affective response feeds back to trigger an amplified experience of danger. Additionally, voluntary choices made under the influence of EMPs are often the causes of suffering that can bring a client to therapy. In the "ABC model" of CBT therapy where "Adversities" interact with "Beliefs" to cause "Consequences," This suffering arises from "C" for Consequences.

With the example of Margaret later in the chapter, we'll see how the result of having a dull and uninteresting life turned out to be the consequence of an inner strategy of self-effacement, originally designed to protect her from her father's criticism. In that way, her EMP led indirectly to her chief complaint. Consequences can be far-reaching, extending beyond families to social groups and to human systems, small, large, and even worldwide.

THE INNER WORKINGS OF EMPS

How Do We Know About Them?

The main body of work regarding the inner workings of EMPs has been in the area of learned fear response (Ledoux, 2016). There, experiments with different mammals as well as humans have shown the same basic brain systems operating in closely analogous ways. This is fortunate and remarkably helpful for us. It is unusual to find an animal model that is not just an analogue, but as true an example as the human one. In this case, the thoroughly studied paradigm of the learned fear response provides an example of an EMP, found equally in humans and other mammals.

In learned fear experiments, a painful or noxious stimulus, such as an electric shock, is associated with a neutral one, such as ringing a bell. The individual quickly learns that the bell predicts a shock and responds with self-protective behavior. Next, the bell is rung but is no longer accompanied by a shock. For a while, the individual continues to react *as if* the shock is still about to take place. These responses are no longer appropriate, nor are they adaptive, which makes them a perfect fit for the definition of an EMP. They are entrenched, that is, not easy to change, they are maladaptive since they are no longer needed, and they are recognizable, repetitive patterns.

The most interesting part of the research, for our purposes, is how the fear response can be eliminated. We'll see below that only two mechanisms have been identified as capable of downgrading and eliminating the fear response. Both have been studied extensively, and interestingly, we'll see that those two change mechanisms are set in motion by elements present in essentially every psychotherapy.

Not All EMPs Originate in the Amygdala

Fear responses originate mainly in the amygdala, but they are not the only threat-processing survival circuits relevant to psychotherapy. The work of Jaak Panksepp (2012) shows that other subcortical (limbic) threat processing systems are also important but involve different anatomical structures and use different neurotransmitters. For example, the PANIC/GRIEF system, focused on the threat of losing a vital relationship, is located in different structures, particularly the anterior cingulate, and utilizes several different neurotransmitters. For our purposes, these diverse threat processing centers are more the same than different. When we look at them from the point of view of the flow of information, each has a threat detection schema, a warning signal/nonconscious emotion, and a response selection schema. That's why we are generalizing about all of the brain's threat-processing systems, rather than treating the EMPs arising from each structure as separate. The action of psychotherapy is the same for all of them, and, while waiting for further research confirmation, it is clinically useful to presume they all follow the same steps as outlined above.

The Flow of Information

Figure 6.1 shows the flow of information for any survival circuit and its threat processing function.

As the diagram shows, information flows into the basic inner mind from the outside environment and from within, including from consciousness. That data is appraised at multiple levels, but the final determination is shown within the dark survival circuit block. First, the threat detection schema performs pattern matching to predict that a danger is imminent. Next, the warning signal consisting of nonconscious emotion lets the rest of the brain know a threat has been detected and that a response is required. From there, the response selection schema is activated and assembles a protective response corresponding to the details of the threat. Of the five paths that link information to action, two direct pathways activate the autonomous bodily embodiments of the response, including affect. Meanwhile, the three indirect elements, thoughts, feelings, and

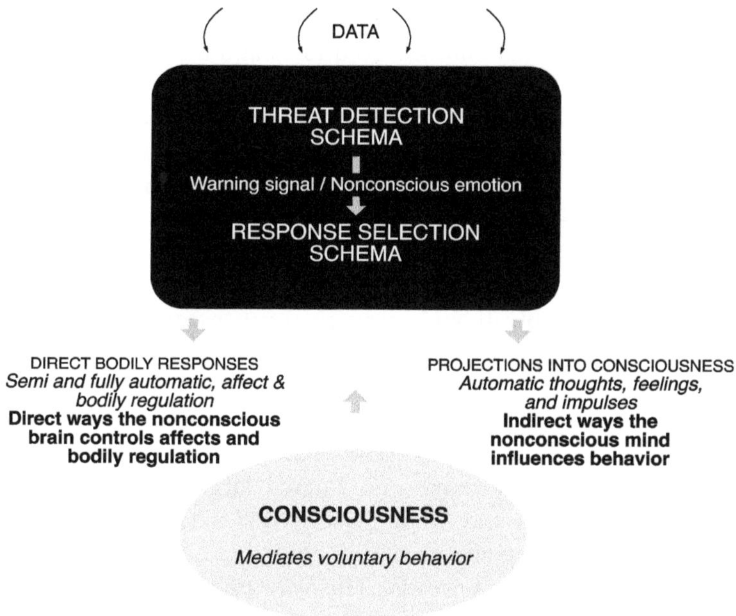

Figure 6.1 Outputs of the Basic Inner Mind

impulses are projected into consciousness, where they exert strong influences on conscious experience and decision-making. Looking at the diagram for points of intervention, the two schemas, the threat detection schema and the response selection schema, will turn out to be prime targets where psychotherapy can modify the logic leading to the outward expression of an EMP.

LEARN TO THINK LIKE THE INNER MIND

In doing clinical work, as we explore how to visualize what's happening in the inner mind, it is also helpful to imagine how the inner mind thinks. In this section, we look at how the inner mind, in contrast to conscious thought, processes information in nonverbal form. We'll also see how it works with that information to answer questions like whether there is a threat and what to do about it.

Information: "Anything That Can Be Described in Poetry"

In considering the associative thinking of the inner mind, we need to look first at the form of information it operates with. To the inner mind, information means chunks of meaning that have associations. A word, a feeling, a color, an image, a vibe, all are held as chunks of information and associated with other chunks. To understand this, we need to know how information is stored in the brain.

Eric Kandel won the Nobel Prize for discovering how information is encoded (2007). He showed that information is represented by groups of neurons that fire together. They do so because of the strength of the synapses that connect them. Those groups of neurons, then, can represent any kind of thing. In this way, groups of neurons that tend to fire together can represent any chunk of information under the sun. This process is an incredibly flexible way to store information. The inner mind doesn't need to store things in categories; it simply attaches associations. That's why we can easily think of related words. They arise from nonconscious places in the mind where *things*, that is, chunks of information, can have any and all kinds of associations.

This is where poetry comes in. Poetry largely ignores logic and puts words together in ways that don't always make literal sense. Our inner mind is comfortable with that and uses associations to make meaning out of the poet's words. The way poetry describes meaning through associations and connotation is very similar to the native way information is handled in the inner mind. Words in poetry are like chunks of information in the inner mind. In fact, a good way to define what can be stored in the inner mind is *anything that can be described in poetry.* That can include the varied things already mentioned, as well as things like a weird feeling, a fashion look, or a feeling about the future. The categories are unlimited, and the contents can be absolutely anything, anything that can be described in poetry.

How Does the Inner Mind Come to Logical Conclusions?

Poetry is all about metaphor, representing one thing by its association with something else. That is how the inner mind handles all kinds of relationships between chunks of information. In 1918, the New York Tribune first mentioned the proverb, "It's not what you know, but who you know." Perhaps that's a way to describe the inner mind's chunks of information. They are, in large part, defined by their associations. That's why metaphor is the inner mind's most natural way of describing something: "It's like..." In contrast to conscious logic, the inner mind doesn't concern itself with the precise nature of a relationship. A color might be associated with a feeling or a word with its connotation.

This simple system of associations allows for nonconscious logic, in which one thing stands for another. This implies an if-then logic that is perfect for pattern matching, especially because it is fuzzy: it gives strong and weak connections between things that are more or less the same. It is fast and practical, but not precise. Formal, conscious logic is much more exact. Having both kinds of logic, fuzzy associations and sharp distinctions helps humans to function smoothly. Imagine how difficult life would be if we only had one of the two systems?

Physiologically, groups of neurons representing different things tend to fire together; that's how the brain keeps track of associations. We can visualize clumps of connected neurons lighting up and, in turn, lighting up other clumps where the two meanings have some kind of association.

It's helpful also to realize that associations can be stronger or weaker, depending on the strength of the synapses that connect the neurons.

Not all associations are positive. The brain is quite capable of making negative associations in the form, *if this, then not that.* Think of how rapidly and naturally the mind comes up with the opposite of a word or concept. On the other hand, as Freud astutely pointed out, the inner mind does not have a native concept for the absence of something. To test this, we need only try telling a small child that monsters don't exist. It simply won't compute.

To understand how the inner mind thinks, we can contrast these simple associations with the much more precise relationships the conscious mind uses in its logic. There, we care whether two things are identical or merely similar. "Are they identical or fraternal twins?" Conscious logic cares about the differences between *identical* and *similar* or between *similar* and *vaguely related.* We evaluate a student's intelligence with questions to test the ability to understand subtle relationships, like "True or False: Fish is to Water as Bird is to Air?" For more about this, see Namburi et al. (2015).

Information Processing in Survival Circuits

Work on the fear system has shown that threat identification is done through "predictive coding," a nonlinear process of matching inputs to expectations on multiple levels of abstraction. Nonlinear means it doesn't go step by step, but repeatedly tests out expectations against inputs, looking at the closeness of fit, and making adjustments with each trial to reduce "prediction error." The same form of pattern matching logic that works for identifying threats is also used for identifying objects. Most of us have experienced this when we misidentified someone or something at a distance, based on what we were *expecting,* then realized our brain's error.

At a brain level, the logic of the inner mind is very basic, consisting of simple pattern matching through predictive coding. This information processing is fast, but not always accurate. Due to evolution's understandable emphasis on survival, the mind would rather err on the side of over-identifying threats rather than under-identifying them. We can see this in the way clients generalize from one or a few bad experiences. A warning signal/nonconscious emotion is often produced for situations that are only distantly related to actual experiences.

While we are visualizing clumps of interconnected neurons, I should point out that they are not necessarily located physically close to one another. From the point of view of the flow of information, what's essential is that synapses join them together functionally, even though they might be spread out anatomically. Moreover, the details of how information is encoded physically are yet more complex, using fast and slow firing rates. Knowing these details isn't necessary for our purposes, but those who are interested can refer to Wang and Cui (2018).

Some templates of threats are inborn. Research has shown that humans have an inborn fear of snakes. Threats such as being abandoned and alone or facing danger are also inborn and even have their own subcortical real estate. At the same time, a lot of what is identified as threatening comes from experience. Let's say that in the early family life of a client, assertiveness leads to yelling and rejection. Then, loud voices might become associated with the probability of abandonment and would trigger a strong warning signal in the form of a nonconscious emotion.

The response selection schema, the second stage of logic in threat processing, applies stored rules using similar pattern matching and predictive coding to make a detailed match. In the case of the loud voices, the selected behavior pattern might be a response of pleading with the person, "Please don't leave me!" That only makes the situation worse, so it is an EMP, but the information processing behind it uses if-then logic, performed using an association between the details of a threat and a specific combination of response elements. When we say a situation "triggers" a specific problem response, we are talking about just this kind of if-then logic.

Now, with an idea of how this nonconscious logic works, we can picture how it serves the purposes of evolution. Evolution worries first and foremost about survival. The first use of logic is to identify threats to survival. In the case of humans, in contrast to other animals, those threats are largely social ones. Threats are stored as patterns of information, and when there is a match with current inputs, then a warning is activated. The logic is fuzzy because there are different strengths of association.

When a threat is especially dangerous, a wider range of circumstances might trigger a match. The same system can be used for less serious threats and even for opportunities, but the associations might be weaker and less rigid. In each case, the first stage of logic identifies circumstances that require a response. Next, a warning signal/nonconscious emotion indicates the need to respond, and finally, a second stage of logic determines what the response should be. It is useful to think of these as sequential steps, but in truth, they are more likely to be nonlinear.

The All-Important Warning Signal

The warning signal that is the product of the initial threat detection schema is critical because it determines whether a response will be generated at all. As indicated earlier, the warning signal is also a nonconscious emotion or proto-emotion. It is often very revealing to ask clients about the dreaded emotion that triggers their EMP. What they tell us is a translation from the inner mind's nonconscious emotion, but it is often both accurate and revealing.

I mentioned Margaret at the beginning of the chapter as coming to therapy with a chief complaint that her life was dull and boring. As we soon found out, that was because every time she thought of doing something interesting and visible to others, EMPs kicked in to discourage her. We will use her case going forward to see how we can apply our understanding of EMPs in a real-life situation.

We knew she felt discouraged from within when she thought of doing something interesting or that could bring attention to herself. But seeking yet more accurate empathy, one day I asked, "What exactly does your mind dread that could happen if you don't take to heart your father's criticisms that you had nothing to offer and that no one would be interested in anything you might produce?" Suddenly, tears came, indicating affective activity originating in the inner mind. This was entirely automatic, and she was a bit embarrassed. I gave her a few moments. Then I asked her what those tears might have meant. To both of our surprise, she immediately answered that she would be ostracized from the family and no longer feel like she belonged there or anywhere.

Instantaneously, we were both aware that the family she was talking about had long since disappeared and that her current family, herself and her husband, was a comfortable place where she really did belong. What we both heard, coming up as a translation into words of what her inner mind was warning about, was a very specific nonconscious emotion. The inner version of this emotion not only shapes her response but also

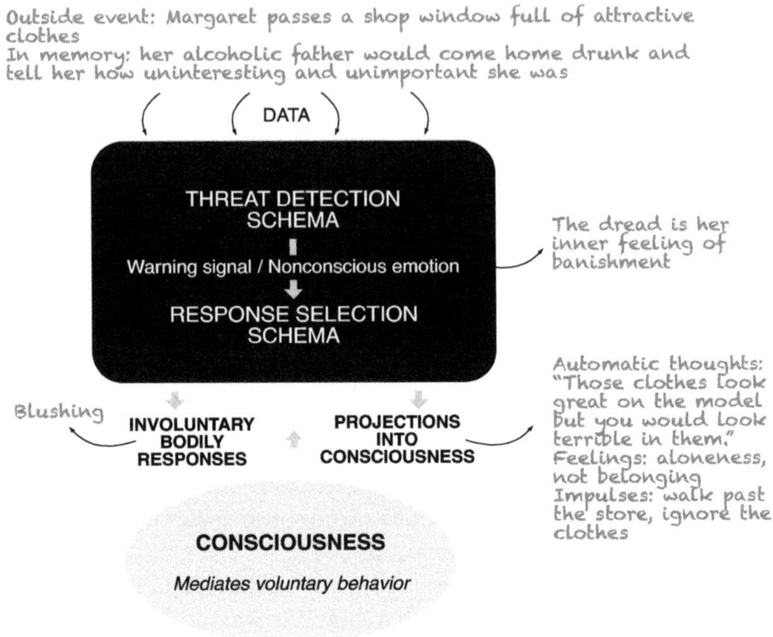

Figure 6.2 Margaret's Bottom Level EMP

shows how her inner mind remained frozen in time, reacting to fears from long ago.

The Importance of Nonconscious Emotion

The fact that the warning signal is not generic, but a specific emotion tied to particular circumstances, gives it great value for gaining understanding and accurate empathy. We'll see in Chapter 10 how that understanding will also help us find new, disconfirming information to replace the old logic of Margaret's schemas. That kind of transformational change will help her, from the bottom up, no longer to adopt self-deprecating responses in order to protect herself from being banished from her former family.

As discussed in Chapter 4, we can think of the inner mind, the subcortical, limbic brain, as the source of unconscious precursor emotions. The word emotion comes from Latin, for *out* and *move*. Emotions are what move us to do things. They make the dog growl. They make Margaret cry, and they are translated into her conscious mind to give words for the painful and upsetting conscious feeling that she could lose her family.

When we look at this from the point of view of the inner mind's mission to protect, it seems quite natural. Nonconscious emotion is the signal that launches responses, including EMPs. Those responses can remain completely nonconscious, or they can set off bodily reactions like tears. They can also function as precursors to conscious thoughts and feelings, like Margaret's feeling of loss about being banned from her family. To state this succinctly:

> *The identification of a threat is done through associative logic, and that conclusion is represented by activation of a warning signal consisting of a nonconscious emotion. That warning triggers selection of a response, which is then manifested in the form of bodily changes and conscious experiences.*

At this point, we have a visual map of how the inner mind handles threats and produces EMPs. What is remarkable is that this understanding, based on the flow of information, shows how much all EMPs have in common and how we can consider them as a group, even though in life they cover a vast and varied range. We also have some sense of how information, as it is stored and processed in the inner mind, is quite different from our conscious notions of information. From here, let's move toward understanding the strategies the inner mind uses to power EMPs. Before we do that, we need to look at a quirk in the functioning of survival circuits in general.

SURPRISE: EMPS AIM TO KILL THE MESSENGER

We might naturally think that the goal of EMPs is survival, but that is not quite true. The brain has evolved for survival and procreation of the species, but the operation of the inner mind takes a shortcut. EMPs are designed to quiet the warning signal rather than to seek the actual elimination of danger. As long as the two goals are in sync, the system works perfectly.

The warning signal is the brain's only representation of danger and functions as a kind of *proxy* for it. The aim of an EMP is to suppress the warning signal/nonconscious emotion, rather than the danger itself. This is much more efficient than having the mind repeatedly assess the danger to determine if the response is working. Instead, it checks to see if the warning signal is less intense. In lower mammals, that works quite well. If the danger is a predator and the options are fight, flight, or freeze, the choices are well-suited to maximize survival, and it's not too hard for the inner mind's schemas to calculate the best one for the circumstances. The social nature of human life adds infinite complexity as well as opportunities for error.

Especially in humans, the goal of quieting the warning signal can lead to results that diverge drastically from what is best for survival. Among survivors of trauma, the client who uses drugs to escape memories of trauma is doing nothing to improve safety or survival. Any reminder of the trauma will activate their threat detection schema and its product, the warning signal/nonconscious emotion. The response is aimed solely at avoiding the pain of remembering. This makes sense because the warning signal/nonconscious emotion is the inner mind's primary way of representing the danger itself. They are related, but not always identical. It is not surprising, especially given the complexity of human life, that avoiding the dreaded nonconscious emotion is not always the same as avoiding the original danger.

A dramatic example is suicide. If the dreaded nonconscious emotion is due to the prediction of a threat, then suicide does nothing for survival but does kill the messenger responsible for the unbearable pain.

In working with clients, as we will see in the next chapter, it is much more productive to ask about the dreaded nonconscious emotion than about the danger itself. For Margaret, it was the feeling of losing her place in the family.

Now it's time to look at how inner selves go about softening the inner warning signal that they so dread.

SOME STRATEGIES INNER SELVES ADOPT

Inner selves make use of a dizzying range of strategies. What they have in common is that they all represent ways to eliminate or diminish a dreaded nonconscious emotion. This is a *negative feedback loop*, a common means of stabilizing any system. The home thermostat is an example of such a negative feedback loop. It turns off the heat when it gets too warm. Similarly, EMPs represent strategies for turning off the warning that sets them in motion. Here are some examples of the mind's rich collection of approaches.

Simple avoidance: Trauma survivors often avoid reminders that might activate painful emotions and bring them to consciousness.

Avoidance by dissociation: The inner mind makes use of the inborn ability to dissociate to avoid recall of painful events, to prevent incompatible experiences from colliding, and to distance itself from intolerable distress.

Avoidance by drug and alcohol use: These can dull or eliminate the impact, even awareness, of negative nonconscious emotions.

Turning passive to active: Clients enact destructive behaviors through their own will and control instead of having painful acts done to them.

Avoidance by opposite emotions: Anger can block the experience of pain and grieving, while sadness can block anger.

Blocking emotional processing: Grieving is normally self-healing, but can be kept out of consciousness, blocking progress toward healing. Anger, too, can be kept out of consciousness where it remains alive and unresolved.

Opposing painful truths about the self: The inner mind can use action as well as words to express the opposite of a source of pain. Examples are exaggerated physical strength, needing nothing or no one, and overdoing other desirable attributes. Messages expressed in words or action can be designed to compete with sources of direct pain as well as self-inflicted shame.

Allaying guilt by deserving punishment: Nonconscious guilt can be calmed by performing immoral actions leading to self-condemnation and/or real punishment.

Projection and other cognitive distortions: Cognitive strategies shift responsibility and, with them, potential guilt or shame.

Internalizing values as deterrents: Values like pride in being tough can function as deterrents to neediness or passive tendencies, which then prevent shame.

Hypervigilance and bracing: An unspoken state of tension is maintained to create the inner illusion of readiness for anticipated hurt or vulnerability.

Simple denial: The act of thinking, saying, or expressing in acting the opposite of an uncomfortable idea.

Denial by idealization or denigration: Asserting a perception opposite to the dreaded one.

Denial by rationalization: Using cognitive distortions and rationalizations to deny dreaded facts or justify unhealthy actions.

Attitudes and values that normalize the abnormal: Seeing oneself as unworthy can, for example, serve to shift pain due to the abnormal behavior by a parent.

Anxiety and panic attacks: These are inborn tendencies of the inner mind that have the effect of influencing the conscious mind toward being prepared for a catastrophe by projecting scary metaphors into consciousness. Cognitive distortions like catastrophization further amplify the influence.

Depression: A presumably inborn survival mechanism, likely aimed at conserving resources to increase survival, is launched when the inner self predicts failure.

Bodily symptoms: Can embody and express nonconscious emotions that have been blocked from healthy conscious expression.

Obsession as pseudo-solution: Obsessing is a partially inborn way to cope with insoluble problems by incessantly thinking or acting in ways that give the illusion of dealing with them.

Keeping hope alive: Acceptance is painful and hard. Many strategies support false hope in order to avoid having to acknowledge or accept a failure or loss.

Seeking what was missed: Painful acceptance of a shortfall can be avoided by seeking gifts, attention, or tokens from other persons or sources seen as substitutes for what was missed.

Those are some of the very many strategies embodied in EMPs to quell the inner mind's warning signals/nonconscious emotions.

With this picture in mind of how EMPs operate, we're ready to dig into the work of psychotherapy. In the next chapter, we'll have a change of pace as we discover Five Key Questions, where pursuing accurate empathy will not only strengthen the therapeutic relationship but will also allow memory reconsolidation to bring about enduring change.

Key Points

- Every EMP consists of a threat detection schema, a warning signal consisting of a nonconscious emotion, a response selection schema, a combination of direct bodily effects and indirect conscious experiences of thoughts, feelings, and impulses, as well as the consequences they lead to.
- The immediate goal of EMPs is to avoid or diminish the nonconscious experience of dreaded negative nonconscious emotions.
- In EMPs, each of the two direct and three indirect outputs of the inner mind has important effects on the client's life. These are best illustrated when conscious intentions are the opposite of the inner mind's plans, as in addictions and with compulsive behaviors.
- The learned fear research paradigm is the source of much of what is known about threat processing and how outdated responses can be changed.

- Information is encoded in the brain in free-form, unstructured chunks of associated neurons that tend to fire together. The implicit learning we are concerned with is nonverbal and associative in nature and can hold anything that can be described in poetry.
- Nonconscious logic, or predictive coding, matches patterns to make decisions.
- EMPs utilize a wide variety of strategies to avoid activating negative nonconscious emotions associated with threats. These can be detected as affects and sometimes verbalized by clients in conscious words.

REFERENCES

Ecker, B., Ticic, R., & Hulley, L. (2024). *Unlocking the emotional brain: Memory reconsolidation and the psychotherapy of transformational change.* Taylor & Francis.

Kandel, E. R. (2007). *In search of memory: The emergence of a new science of mind.* W. W. Norton & Company.

Ledoux, J. (2021). As soon as there was life, there was danger: the deep history of survival behaviours and the shallower history of consciousness. *Philosophical Transactions of the Royal Society B: Biological Sciences, 37,* 20210292.

Ledoux, J., & Pine, D. (2016). Using neuroscience to help understand fear and anxiety: A two-system framework. *The American Journal of Psychiatry, 173*(11), 1083–1093.

Namburi, P., Beyeler, A., Yorozu, S., Calhoon, G., Halbert, S., Wichmann, R., Holden, S., Mertens, K., Anahtar, M., Felix-Ortiz, A., Wickersham, I., Gray, J., & Tye, K. (2015). A circuit mechanism for differentiating positive and negative associations. *Nature, 520,* 675–678.

Panksepp, J., & Biven, L. (2012). *The archaeology of mind: Neuroevolutionary origins of human emotions (Norton series on interpersonal neurobiology).* W. W. Norton & Company.

Wang, J. H., & Cui, S. (2018). Associative memory cells and their working principle in the brain. *F1000Research,* 7, 108.

CHAPTER 7

Five Key Questions: A Method for Seeking Accurate Empathy

Thinking of the main job of the therapist as seeking accurate empathy, these questions are a good way to make it happen. Accurate empathy will help build a strong and trusting relationship and will give you a window into details of the client's EMPs that are crucial for achieving enduring and transformative change. It is useful in sessions, but also as an aid to formulating cases in supervision and other settings. This is not the only way to conduct therapy, but it is simple, easy to remember, and compatible with diverse therapeutic techniques and traditions.

How Seeking Answers Can Lead to Change

Just as accurate empathy means seeking a deepening, emotionally engaged understanding, the five questions are a guide to a progressively deeper understanding rather than a definitive answer or label. No one wants to be labeled, but just about everyone wants to be understood. That means an answer that categorizes or labels, such as, "Oh, you are angry!" won't be satisfying. Instead, we seek a deepening understanding of the background and present circumstances that trigger an EMP, as well as how its protective strategy works. Furthermore, engaging with the client in seeking understanding together is part of what strengthens trust in the relationship. At the same time, our exploration of the details will be heard and felt deep in the subcortical inner mind, where our target schemas are held. As we get close to problem areas, we'll notice affect, our sign that the relevant schemas have become neurologically active, and that, we will soon learn, is the first requirement for enduring change in the specifics of the client's EMP.

DOI: 10.4324/9781003619659-8

When affect comes into the room, that is the first sign that the inner mind is sensing a threat and is in the process of launching a response. Affect is the fastest and most direct response. It is also the most unmistakably authentic because it is not under voluntary control. That's why therapists are especially attuned to bodily changes like tears or breathing that are among the inner mind's direct responses to danger. There is a reason why in-session emotion is one of the common factors associated with therapeutic success. It's because those emotions reflect activation of the inner mind's warning signal/nonconscious emotion, and that tells us there is an opening for change.

The process of seeking accurate empathy works far better when the client feels safe. That is one of the main functions of the other common factors, the ones involving trust in the therapist and the process. Not only does a good relationship facilitate communication with the deep subcortical inner mind, but it also provides support for the client to take emotional risks and try scary new behaviors.

There is more. We want to set up a collision between the old schemas and new information, a collision that will lead to rewriting the ways the mind appraises a threat and chooses a response. Making it easier for the client to say out loud how the inner mind thinks is a good way to begin preparing for such a collision. That's because the conscious logical mind is listening. It hears the inner mind's outdated logic and can send messages down to the subcortical brain that there is a better way. The new information disconfirms the old, and that turns out to be a key to enduring change.

Imagine a client who is afraid of being assertive. He explains, "Yes, that's right, I feel an internal truth that if I'm assertive, I'll be severely punished." Just the fact of stating such a deeply felt internal truth will be met by an equally clear conscious awareness that those punishments are a thing of the past, and there is no longer any reason to be afraid. The contradiction will be transmitted and heard deep down. We can be confident of that because, at that moment, affect tells us there is an open communication channel. As the next chapter on change mechanisms will explain, a prediction error will be generated, the old schema will be rewritten, and the old EMP will have lost its reason for existing. It doesn't always happen that neatly and totally, but often it does. That is what is meant by transformative change. Now let's look at the questions, one at a time.

THE FIVE KEY QUESTIONS

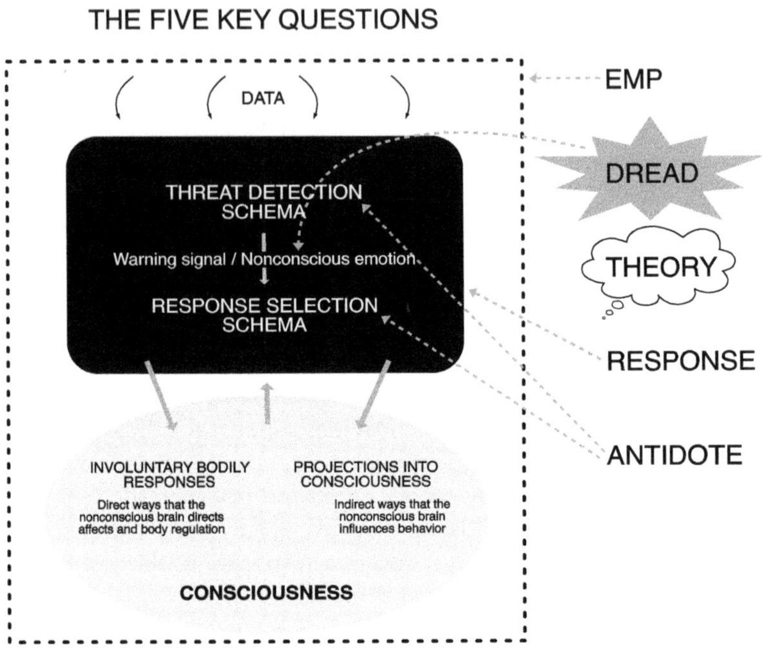

Figure 7.1 Five Key Questions

Question 1. What EMP Is Causing Trouble?

This question is a bit more complex than it might appear. We always want to start with an understanding of the pain that brings the client to therapy. Achieving this understanding in depth isn't always obvious. My very first client said, "I'm not happy." What did that mean? With some people, a simple nudge will start the flow: "Please say more." With others, some teaching may be required: "I hear that, but it's pretty broad. I'd really like to understand what that feels like and when it started. When was the last time you felt happy?"

Any time we seek accurate empathy about an EMP, we need to listen for the entrenchment that has prevented the client from changing. Along with that, positive psychology says it is important to understand strengths and positive attributes that will help the client overcome entrenchment and may serve to replace the old response When we use accurate empathy to understand strengths, acknowledging them out loud helps clients "own" them and have more confidence in using the resilience they already have.

We are going to need a really good understanding of the source of pain to see how an EMP leads to the outward trouble. Margaret complained that her life was dull and unsatisfying. It took a while to understand that the dullness was because each time she thought of doing something interesting, her inner mind would tell her that she had nothing to offer and no one would want to see anything she produced. Her EMP was an example of identifying with the aggressor; she was adopting her father's critical attitude toward herself to make sure she stayed in his good graces. It was drastically outdated, since her father had died some years earlier, and she had married a thoroughly appreciative man. Once the connection between boredom and her inner fear was established, it became rather simple to understand her lowest layer of EMP. The next example is more typical in that it involves three layers of EMPs.

For Alan, a retired corporate lawyer, the top layer EMP was to be drunk for days on a destructive bender. This had been triggered recently when his performance was less than stellar on the golf course. He had worked hard in counseling and had made some headway with top-down (willpower) efforts to change his drinking behavior, but kept being triggered into drinking bouts, each one more dangerous than the last. But why such an extreme reaction to doing poorly in golf? His attitude toward success was dysfunctional, too, pointing to another layer of EMP. He had to succeed at everything and had to let everyone know. Eventually, the explanation came out. The second layer was that he had to succeed at everything in order to compensate for feeling very bad about himself. And those bad feelings arose from a third layer of EMP. It wasn't so clear quite what that layer was.

Like Margaret, he, too, had been viciously criticized by a stepfather. His lowest level of EMP was internalizing his stepfather's impossible standards and criticizing himself. By putting himself down, he gained some safety because neither his stepfather nor anyone else could get to him first. We worked with that idea, but it didn't clear things up. He had yet another bender. There had to be something bigger.

Yes, there was a more troubling reason for feeling ashamed of himself. After some years of off-and-on therapy, he was ready for us to get to this layer and question the shame he was now able to acknowledge. In his therapy, we needed to create a collision between an inner "truth" that he was a shameful failure and the real truth, that he was an imperfect but caring and generous human being. We did, and the result was transformative change. I'll tell the rest of the story when we get to question number 5.

These examples will serve to show that understanding the relevant EMP is far from trivial. It may take time to work our way toward an answer, which may still turn out to have additional twists and turns. At the outset, there was no way to understand the full architecture of Alan's three layers of EMP. It was only possible to work with the first layer and remain open to understanding the next one. The better we understand, the more we feel empathy for the young selves who long ago had to cope alone with terrible hurt. Not only that, but Alan had learned to blame the wrong person, himself, both as a child and in adulthood, holding himself in contempt for failing to stop drinking and for not performing at golf.

Question 2. What Inner DREAD Is Being Avoided?

Dread is a highly evocative word to describe the inner warning signal/nonconscious emotion we have talked so much about. We don't know what nonconscious emotions feel like, but the inner mind is good at translating them into words to help us understand those deep feelings and their context in detail. It is the communication channel between the inner mind and consciousness that makes it possible and productive to ask the question. Asking is a bit tricky because, not infrequently, the conscious mind will intercept the question and want to handle it by digging, that is, by trying intellectually to deduce the answer using conscious logic and memory. Unfortunately, doing that will automatically close the channel to the inner mind, so it is better to catch intellectualization early and try to help the client let go and quit "trying too hard." We may have to teach them to relax and let their inner mind do the work.

The answer may or may not come directly. It helps to listen for it in some form we may not have expected. If affect appears, we have won the lottery. That usually means a channel is open, both to and from the inner mind. Sharing our own thoughts can sometimes help if we are not pushy. Our goal is to hear whether our guess resonates, meaning the client experiences a feeling of truth. It is also acceptable to try to infer from indirect evidence, as long as we respect the degree of uncertainty in our conjecture.

As I've pointed out before, a question asked in session will be heard by the inner mind as an unfinished story. The human mind is highly drawn to knowing the ending or outcome, and that is probably the same as our need to find the answer to a question. Both tap into the same instinct as our need for closure. This characteristic makes asking a question a lot like planting a seed. Even if it does not germinate immediately, we can expect it to create an inner tension until an answer is found.

I often find myself saying something like this to a client: "What is the deep-down emotion that your mind is dreading?" or "What is the emotion that your inner mind is trying so hard to keep at bay?"

Richard, a 74-year-old retired banker, has been depressed for about a month. He was admitted to the inpatient psychiatric service after his wife stopped him from jumping off the balcony of his apartment. In the history he gave, he said he had been fired from his job a few years earlier, had been experiencing vision and hearing loss, and had recently lost his brother to a heart attack. The outward manifestation of his top-level EMP is clear enough: seriously trying to end his life. But what is the dread that would have been avoided by jumping?

With Richard safely in the hospital, we will need to explore thoughtfully and carefully, listening and looking for signs of affect. There is a good chance that the few things he has volunteered will lead to an understanding of the nonconscious emotion, the dread driving his suicidal EMP. We might be tempted to say it is the combination of all the adverse experiences he has encountered, but that would be premature and pure conjecture. Besides, it is too general. Understanding the specifics is what is therapeutic. That's how we seek accurate empathy. For example, if I hear two reasons for something, that means I'm getting an abstraction, a composite of the two, so I nudge by asking for only one, the one that is most important right now. In seeking accurate empathy, *evidence-based* means having the patience to keep listening until we can confirm that something is stirring inside. Usually, there is just one thing, one aspect of experience that comes closest to the precise dread. What clinches the answer is affect appearing at the exact moment the source of dread becomes apparent. That's what happened when Richard explained how his brother's death made him see himself hurtling down a path toward the end of his own life. It was a turning point for him, just to share the dread of his own deterioration and death.

But the dread element in an EMP, the negative, nonconscious emotion, is supposed to be something unrealistic. It's supposed to be an inner truth that turns out not to be true so we can help install a more truthful version. Correct. What was unrealistic about Richard's dread was not the literal truth but the degree. For children, death is unthinkable. It's something that *must not happen*. Healthy adults grow into the ability to accept the inevitability of the end of life. Without getting into the debate about how much suffering is acceptable at the end of life, Richard's horror, the abruptness of his decision, and the violence of the death he sought suggested a childlike intensity to his feeling. I did not have the privilege of knowing the end of the story, but it is likely that, with more sharing of his deep angst, his initial inability to face the end of life will change as he grows into accepting his life on its terms.

This example illustrates a helpful principle when listening for the dread. It is asking oneself if the emotion is out of proportion with the current adult situation. Smaller children have bigger emotions. When I see such emotions, I ask myself, "At what age would this emotion be appropriate?" That often leads to the original circumstance and the original dread that an EMP was designed to avoid. It also highlights how the problem is the absoluteness of a dread, not its literal truth.

I'm sure you are thinking that having practice is helpful when seeking answers to these questions. It is, but it's also important not to worry when answers are not clear. Just seeking together helps build a trusting partnership, but, more importantly, it may be too soon for the answer to come. We need to have patience. Besides that, as we learned in Chapter 1, it's important to pay attention to what we don't know. This question also shows why supervision, experience, and receiving client feedback are all part of continually growing as a therapist.

Question 3. What Is Your THEORY or Working Hypothesis About How this EMP Got Established and How It Is Triggered?

Going back again to the first chapter, always having a working hypothesis makes one a better observer. It sets you and your own inner mind on a quest for clues to confirm or disconfirm your theory. This question may be more for the therapist to think about than to ask the client. As it becomes clearer, sharing may become more useful for the relationship and the work. My experience is that making psychotherapy mysterious does not impart any extra benefits, while sharing can lead to unexpected insights. As a result, I'm more likely to share an idea even if it may not be fully ripe.

Of course, it is important not to become too attached to our theory. We should rejoice when we discover a hypothesis is wrong, because then we will learn something new and important that we didn't expect. With this question, we are building a tentative theory about a serious problem that caused the inner mind to dig into its resources for the best protective response it could muster. It is interesting to guess about the age and circumstances. We need to picture the circumstances as perceived by the inner mind, not necessarily what an adult observer might see or even the real truth.

Here is an example of a hypothesis where the question is whether it is based on perception or reality. Liz's adult children have shown strong signs of feeling they didn't get enough mothering from their professional mom. Liz was my client, and it was clear that her own EMP consisted in part of constantly feeling guilty about not giving more to others. Our hypothesis was that she grew up with internal values that demanded she be totally attentive to the needs of others while neglecting her own needs. As a result, she constantly felt as if she had not given enough to her children. In reality, she appeared to have been quite attentive but often expressed out loud how she felt guilty for not giving enough. The children may have picked up her feelings and felt, incorrectly but genuinely, that they were deprived.

My hypothesis regarding the children's sense of deprivation is that she actually took good care of the children but transmitted to them the sense that it was never enough. This could have given them the subjective impression of being deprived when they may actually have received a healthy amount of attention. Am I certain? No, I'm still open to the possibility that my interpretation may not have been correct.

Question 4. What Is the New RESPONSE to Replace the EMP?

This question looks at the second stage of logic in the inner mind, the response selection schema, where the choice is made of what protective response to launch. Changing this logic means replacing it through memory reconsolidation with a more desirable response taken from the client's repertoire of available options. Finding a better response may be obvious, for example, in trauma, no response at all to a formerly frightening experince may be the idea response. On the other hand, a response that is meaningful and feels right to the client may be an adaptation of an existing skill from some other area of experience or it may be a response that has to be learned from scratch. It is often helpful to have a role model or avatar who represents the improved attitude or manner.

Margaret revealed her choice of response in an interesting way. She was thinking about another part of her EMP, manifested by giving too much to her entitled mother-in-law. She felt trapped with no choice but, once more, to go out of her way and do something for the ungrateful woman, knowing she would feel used and unappreciated. Suddenly, she had a feeling, maybe a vision, an inner sense, that she could be free of the weight of this burden. She was trying to put words to something internal and nonverbal, an alternative to the old rule that, being of little value, she would always have to say yes. A new response pattern had appeared, ready for implementation. The next time her mother-in-law demanded a service, at last, she felt capable of taking a deep breath and saying no. The freedom to refuse removed the heavy weight of having no choice.

A New RESPONSE May Have to Be Learned First

Not infrequently, the inner mind can see only one choice of how to respond. The solution may require new learning, to internalize unfamiliar, but ultimately more satisfactory skills. An important example of an alternative is acceptance. This is often the only healthy choice, but it is a learned skill, not one we are born with. Children appear to be programmed not to accept defeat in their growth, survival, and development. Because acceptance is not an option or because it is too painful, it may be avoided and not learned. In adult life, accepting reality on its terms is often less painful than going through the gyrations needed to avoid facing the truth that things happen over which we have no control. For many clients, acceptance of reality will need to be learned and practiced for it to become available as an alternative to denial in its many forms. In such a case, the learning may be challenging but can be an essential part of the therapy.

Another important source of alternative responses is the client's past experience. In the case of John in Chapter 3, his past experience of following "procedure" at work helped him accept therapy. It is often possible to adapt existing skills rather than the client having to learn a new response, and that is almost always better than starting from scratch.

Behavior change creates new experiences, and new experiences provide disconfirming information. Remember that an experience is encoded in the brain as a chunk of information. Trying out a better response in reality or in imagination is often the most effective way to communicate new information to collide with and disconfirm the inner mind's faulty logic, and that can be a necessary step in changing the response selection schema so it adopts the new pattern as the favored response.

Question 5. What Is the Disconfirming ANTIDOTE?

This is perhaps the most challenging of the five questions. We will discuss it in a lot more detail in Chapter 10. The first four questions set the stage. As affects are brought into the room, verifying that the inner mind has been activated, then it's time for a new, contradictory experience or truth to create a collision deep in the subcortical inner mind. That's the disconfirming new information that generates a prediction error and allows memory reconsolidation to rewrite the outdated schemas.

Disconfirming the First, Threat-Detection Schema

The simplest antidotes are the ones that say there is no threat and that the DREAD need not be feared. That happens mainly in trauma, where circumstances have changed, and what was once feared is no longer possible or relevant. It might be that an ex-soldier has returned from the war and will never go back again, but I have seen the inner mind counter that with, "but I might be at the shopping mall and get caught up in a terrorist incident. Then I would have to be ready to protect my family." The disconfirmation that his military service is finished could not work. There had to be a better one.

That situation was further complicated. The ex-soldier had fully accepted his own death, but the thought of losing his wife or child was far beyond acceptance. His current stance, both consciously and nonconsciously was to put all his energy into preparing to prevent the remote possibility of harm to them, leaving no room to join with them in enjoying life. The reality that saving them in those highly unlikely circumstances was not very realistic, but that realization was of no use. The best alternative was to reach inside where his inner child was stuck in an absolute and trade it for a relative truth where he would take all due precautions while accepting the very, very remote possibility of a tragic event. The most common thing that can disconfirm the determination of a threat and invalidate the need for a response is that the meaning of threat is different in childhood compared to adult life. In other words, acceptance, not an option for the child, now in adult life becomes at least thinkable.

What conveys a more accepting attitude is often not intellectual, and in fact, may be the calm voice and attitude of another. The collision is between the client's desperate feeling and the therapist's nonverbal expression of peace. This is exactly what Leslie Greenberg, the founder of emotion-focused therapy means when he talks about "healing emotion with emotion." The client's upset emotion is disconfirmed by the therapist's calm emotion. Even when we use words, it is their connotative meaning and tone of voice that do the hard work. A phrase I have sometimes used is, "the war is over." For me, and for some clients, this has tremendous evocative power to express that the time of dread and anxiety is done, ended.

A related problem in finding an antidote arises with people who are genetically and biologically excessively anxious. Their inner mind projects metaphors into consciousness to express an inner feeling of constant danger. The client's conscious mind reflects the degree of fear using a metaphorical equivalent—say, driving off a bridge. Suggesting that such a thing is highly unlikely doesn't do anything to disconfirm the fear. It is the *possibility* of driving off the bridge. The calamity is still theoretically possible and justifies the anxiety. In the inner mind, the image of going off a bridge is an accurate metaphor for the internal, unspoken terror. One possible antidote might be that worrying won't help and ruins the person's quality of life, but that isn't very compelling. The best antidote is to disconfirm the childlike, "it must not happen" with a more adult, "things happen in life, and we need to accept that just existing is risky." It helps for the client to understand where the inner anxiety comes from, that it is constitutional and not related to real danger.

A similar antidote for disconfirming the threat detection schema is clinical mindfulness. That's the technique used when a client is immersed in a self-absorbed experience of some painful circumstance. The therapist brings a bigger and calmer perspective, letting the client simultaneously experience both responses. It is a procedure that juxtaposes the childlike, self-centered emotions that are often the inner mind's responses with a more mature, philosophical point of view. When clients express their distress out loud, the presence of a calm witness in touch with a bigger perspective conveys a mindful attitude that collides with the distress and creates a healing experience.

Sometimes we can find a deeper and more specific source of the inner mind's anxiety and find an antidote to that, but anxiety can also be genetic and biological, with little in early experience to explain it or to provide grounds for disconfirmation. In Chapter 10, we'll look more at antidotes to the threat detection schema, but now let's turn to the other schema, the response selection schema.

Disconfirming the RESPONSE Selection Schema

I promised to tell the rest of Alan's story here. He was the lawyer with a history of serious alcoholic benders. His deepest EMP was shame. Coping with his father's criticism was one source, but when working with that didn't bring about transformative change, we began to think there was another reason for feeling shame. It took a lot of work to get there, but one day he was ready. We had known from the beginning that he had been sexually molested by a young adult who was a friend of the family. What happened in the therapy room that day was so quiet and simple that it could easily have been missed. In a few words, he described that, living with his punishing and rageful stepfather, he felt incredibly alone and longed for some comfort. The young family friend had expressed genuine warmth and acceptance. He longed for that and, as the attention gradually turned sexual, it wasn't even painful.

That's all he said, but what we both knew what it meant. As a seven-year-old, when the attention became sexual, in his own young mind, failing to fight back meant he was a participant and fully responsible for accepting it. That was the erroneous source of his terrible shame.

As he spoke the few words to describe what he had experienced, it was clear to his conscious mind that he was not at all responsible. The channel was wide open, and the new information struck home in his inner mind, disconfirming and replacing the old rule that he had to spend his life overcompensating to ward off his terrible shame. The old logic was replaced by empathy for his young self.

The change was immediate and transformational. He has not had a drinking bout since, nor has he had to trumpet his accomplishments.

The *corrective emotional experience* described by Alexander and French (French, 1946) is another version of the same juxtaposition, one that takes place in therapies where the client develops transference. The client expects the therapist to respond in a certain way, and the reality turns out quite different. "I know you are going to discharge me from treatment when I tell you this…" When the therapist smiles and does no such thing, a disconfirming experience has just taken place.

Chapter 10 will be devoted to the many varieties of disconfirming thoughts and experiences. They need to be attuned to the precise specifics of the client's DREAD. Every therapy has techniques that support this. In the last chapter, number 14, we'll look at how diverse therapies incorporate this final element in achieving transformational change.

To Share the Questions with the Client or Not

Sharing answers to these questions as we go along can be done explicitly or embedded quietly in the flow of conversation. They can also be kept to oneself if an answer hasn't yet "jelled" or if the client isn't ready to absorb some piece of information.

In general, I don't believe in keeping thoughts secret. In Victorian times, when much of psychotherapy was first developed, the bias was toward withholding. That's when British orphanages prohibited staff from forming bonds with children out of fear of making them dependent. And it was before Bowlby showed the enormous damage that that policy created. It was also a time when deprivation was considered a good way to generate motivation. The field of psychotherapy is still somewhat influenced by a belief in withholding gratification, but times have largely changed.

Often, it is positively helpful to share the questions and tentative answers overtly with the client. Doing so invites their own curiosity and engagement. We need to be careful not to impose our ideas, as the client's are almost always better. We must also be careful not to get into intellectual or abstract territory, where emotion is filtered out. The aim is to help the client draw us into their world so that we both experience empathy.

My own tendency is not only to share the question, but at some point, to explain how memory reconsolidation works along with its two requirements. Most often, this has the result of enhancing client engagement and not derailing the process.

EDTRA: MAKING THE FIVE KEY QUESTIONS EASY TO REMEMBER

A simple mnemonic is EXTRA, with D, for DREAD, in place of the X. To recap, each one asks, "What is the…"

The Five Key Questions are not the only way to guide the sessions, but they are unique in being tied to the specifics of how the inner mind builds EMPs and how they can be changed through memory reconsolidation. These questions have been helpful as a guide to exploration in therapy sessions, in supervision to guide a growing understanding, and in learning to formulate cases as an aid to navigation.

The chapters that follow are intended to help you apply the five questions or any other technique and to conduct therapy effectively.

What is the...

EMP	Dread	Theory	Response	Antidote
Outward description of the **Entrenched Maladaptive Pattern** (**EMP**) of behavior or experience causing client distress?	Dreaded unconscious proto-emotion that signals threat, triggers affect, and that the EMP is designed to avoid or soften?	Working hypothesis to explain the original problem, how it was addressed by the EMP, and what activates it now?	An improved automatic response, learned or adapted, to replace the old, outdated and less healthy EMP response?	Antidote: New and surprising information or experience, delivered non-verbally to disconfirm and rewrite old schemas?

Key Points

- One way to guide therapy sessions is consistently seeking to increase accurate empathy. The Five Key Questions, as described in this chapter, amount to a simple, but sophisticated way to organize that task. The answers sought are not final, but incremental steps in the depth of emotionally engaged understanding.
- Question 1 is, "What EMP is causing trouble?" This question takes us from the client's suffering or distress back to an understanding of how the inner mind's problem-solving strategy is impacting the client's life.

- Question 2 is, "What is the DREAD that the EMP strategy is aimed at avoiding?" That dread is the nonconscious emotion that warns of a threat and leads to affects as well as automatic thoughts, feelings, and impulses.
- Question 3 is, "What is your THEORY or hypothesis to explain the origin and triggers of the EMP?" This may be preliminary, but it helps to have a starting point.
- Question 4 is, "What is the RESPONSE that can replace the old choice of EMP?" This is the improved response pattern the client might learn or locate from past experience.
- Question 5 is, "What is the disconfirming ANTIDOTE?" This is what new information or experience, when delivered to the inner mind, will show that the outdated "truth" can be replaced.
- EDTRA stands for the five keys, EXTRA with the X exchanged with D for DREAD.
- These questions can organize the conversation, not necessarily in order, and they can also be useful for supervision and group discussion. In the end, they will increase accurate empathy.

REFERENCE

French, A. (1946). The principle of corrective emotional experience. In F. Alexander, T. M. French, C. L. Bacon, T. Benedek, R. A. Fuerst, & M. W. Gerard (Eds.), *Psychoanalytic therapy: Principles and application* (pp. 66–70). Ronald Press.

CHAPTER 8

Three Mechanisms of Change

We have seen so far that EMPs are invented to cope with serious challenges, then stored as implicit learning in schemas. Those schemas determine first what is dangerous and then what to do about it. They are held mainly in subcortical structures such as the amygdala. Remarkably, and perhaps reassuringly, just three basic mechanisms, all familiar to neurophysiologists, are enough to explain the actions of psychotherapy and, more importantly, to help clients change the way those schemas work.

1. **New learning** helps add new responses to the inner mind's available repertoire.
2. **Extinction** is how the cortex learns to send inhibitory signals to block maladaptive responses without eliminating the underlying warning signal.
3. **Memory reconsolidation** produces enduring modification of schemas, so the response pattern is changed for a given set of circumstances.

These three are *mechanisms* in contrast to *mediators*. Mediators are associated statistically with success, while mechanisms actually explain cause and effect. That means these three mechanisms explain, on a neurophysiological level, how words, nonverbal information, and relationships are able to bring about change to EMPs. Psychotherapy also has important mediators, in particular, the common factors.

Mechanisms versus Mediators

Our three mechanisms not only explain how therapy brings about change, but how and why common factors mediators are beneficial. For

DOI: 10.4324/9781003619659-9

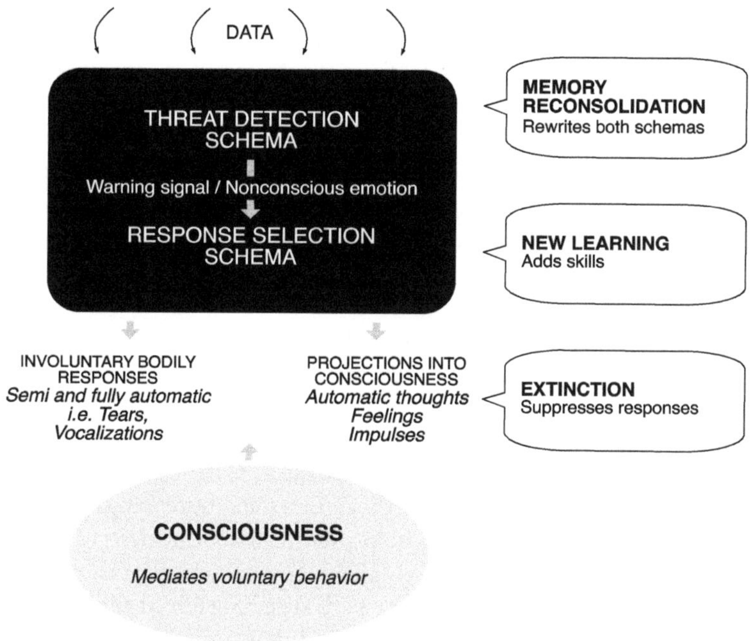

Figure 8.1 Three Change Mechanisms

example, a good relationship helps with the motivation and willingness needed to overcome the entrenchment, that is, the resistance to change, inherent in all EMPs. Trust in the relationship and the process allows the client to accept and benefit from our support as they struggle with inner reluctance to change. With these mechanisms, we can also explain another common factor, the importance of in-session affect, which serves as a marker that a channel is open between the inner mind and consciousness. We need that open channel both to confirm that the relevant schema is in an active state and as a pathway for delivering new, disconfirming information with which to rewrite the schema.

In this discussion, we are focusing on how psychotherapy does its primary job of helping clients change the EMPs responsible for the discomfort that brings them to therapy. There are other, more long-term benefits that have to do with the regulation of hormones, changes in epigenetics, and even the growth of neurons. Those are acknowledged but not emphasized, to allow us to stay focused on precisely how our actions can be instrumental in supporting positive and lasting change.

The Natural Healing of Grief and Anger

There are two processes of self-healing that are often part of psychotherapy. I have mostly left them out of the discussion because all they need is time. They take place automatically if not blocked by avoidance of emotion. Grief is the natural fading of the pain of loss. It can be arrested by avoiding facing the pain, and it can be supported by our witnessing the emotions and recognizing that the time it takes is not in our hands. When grieving is blocked and not progressing, there is an EMP in its way that needs to be explored like other EMPs. The other process is the dissipation of anger. It seems to work the same way, needing to be communicated with a witness, then taking its own time course. The end point is when raging no longer feels like it has any point and it's time to turn to other concerns.

The research on grief and anger is ongoing, so I'll limit what I say to our role in supporting these natural processes. Our job is to help clients articulate their feelings in a way that elicits accurate empathy, to give them the time they need, and to help them not act out destructively. For more detail, I'll leave the reader to check the current literature.

In the remainder of this chapter, we'll discuss each of the three foundational change mechanisms in turn. Each has an important role; however, we will focus last and with the most emphasis on the one I think of as the "Queen of Change Mechanisms," *memory reconsolidation,* because it is the only means psychotherapy has to bring about transformative change. That is, change that is rapid, enduring, and maintained with no further effort. Let's start with *new learning*, the way clients add healthy responses to their available repertoire.

NEW LEARNING

So far in this book, new learning has perhaps not received the attention it deserves. In order to focus on schemas and EMPs, less emphasis has been placed on the ordinary ways humans learn skills and develop what we could call maturity. This is how clients acquire the fourth of the Five Key Questions, the new RESPONSE. EMPs often block new learning and development in ways that limit the options available. Our job as therapists includes helping clients make up for lost ground, so they acquire new skills and adapt old abilities to replace the outdated responses embodied in their EMPs. Thus, new learning and psychological development are very much within the scope of psychotherapy.

One way to appreciate the importance of new learning is to think about how we develop into who we are. The brain is a learning machine, taking in experience and extracting principles to guide us through life. Learning starts in the womb and goes on throughout life.

The kind of learning I'm talking about here is not episodic memory, the type that stores specific experiences. Nor is it the kind that brings back a name or a math fact. The kind we are most interested in is *procedural memory*, for example, how to drink from a glass or what to expect when meeting someone new. It's also referred to as implicit because it is nonconscious. We don't have access to this learning in its native, nonverbal form. Rather, we can only know the contents of procedural memory through what is implied by our outward actions and choices. By implication, we learn about the nonconscious templates that lead to end results. New learning steps in when existing learnings are outdated or maladaptive. It is also how we gain the skills and characteristics that go into psychological development and shape who we are.

New Learning and the Client's Repertoire of Responses

Let's return to John, the man who had a panic attack following the news that he and his wife were pregnant and that he had received a promotion at work. Because of early deprivation and punishment, asking for help went against his values. He was one of those whose inner critic was always watching for signs of weakness and ready to punish with shame. Not only had shame deterred him from even thinking about depending on others, but he had gained no experience in doing so. His EMP was simply not to ask. Beyond shame, he would naturally (due to early learning) assume that the other person would be annoyed at being asked for help and would refuse.

Learning to ask is a skill. It helps to approach the other person with a positive expectation and a sensitivity for how much one is asking. This would not come naturally or easily to John. Typically, those who are expecting a "no" protect themselves by using a tone of voice and language indicating their negative expectation. For helpers who are positively disposed to say "yes," that feels like a lack of appreciation of their willingness and can lead to a negative response, even from a person otherwise quite ready to pitch in.

New learning can be difficult when it comes to practicing new patterns of interaction. Going against automatic defenses and negative expectations is difficult. And yet, the only way to learn and become comfortable and natural with a skill is to try it out and practice repeatedly. What if the initial trial goes badly? Then it requires even more daring and motivation to try again. These are real considerations in psychotherapy. What makes risk-taking worth the stress for John is that, unless he learns the skill, he is doomed to continue living as an island, with the likelihood of further panic attacks, not to mention the wear and tear on a marriage where he has chronically failed to acknowledge or accept gracefully his wife's willing support.

His therapist can help by providing some degree of coaching to encourage him to try and help him experience positive results. That guidance can be critical in helping him add asking for help to his repertoire of available patterns of response. This is a place where CBT has experience that psychodynamically oriented colleagues can learn from.

Making New Learning Easier

In some cases, there is an easier route. At times, the inner mind may leave an available pattern out of its calculations, even though it has been practiced in other contexts. Perhaps at work, John has learned to ask for help, not for his personal needs but because it is required to get the job done. Then an easier way for him to add the new skill will be to leverage his previous experience on the job. Recalling instances of successfully asking for help will give him a template for practicing the new skill of asking for *personal* help. Adapting existing skills is always worth exploring.

New Learning and Psychological Development

Normal psychological development involves an intricate series of learnings that build on top of each other and lead to many of our individual characteristics. That said, the infrastructure of development is new learning, a complex interaction among multiple brain structures, but familiar to all humans (Olsson et al., 2020). Whether it is learning to cross a street safely or how to engage in give and take with others, the patterns involved are internalized by processes that involve intellectual learning, imitation, and practice. When the stakes are high, practicing is often scary and can require some determination. Often, first tries are not graceful; they're even awkward. These experiences are ubiquitous, a part of all of our lives. In the abstract, they seem very simple. But when we look at the specifics, early trials and multiple repetitions are complex and important events in life.

An example relevant to this discussion might be impulse control. Young children learn some degree of impulse control, but that skill becomes more important in early adolescence. That's when kids discover that they must do a boring homework assignment when they'd rather be out with friends or looking at a screen. It is also the skill that allows holding back when it's helpful to do so in a social conversation. This, along with many other skills and habits, makes up the ways we interact with others and with the world. Some people have an easy time with this, and others do not. Especially in the presence of ADHD (Attention Deficit Hyperactivity Disorder), an impulsive adolescence tends to put the individual significantly behind their peers through lack of social competence and difficulty engaging in long hours of practice. That is a common example of a specific area of troubled development.

Psychotherapy Promoting Growth and Maturation

While most of what is written here is about changing maladaptive patterns, a large part of the work that needs to be done in psychotherapy is addressing areas of delayed or arrested growth and development. Here are three other remarkable facts about psychological and emotional development:

1. New learning is not only the mechanism for acquiring any new skill; it is the backbone of psychological development. It works the same as John's development of the skill of asking for support described above.
2. Arrested development can be picked up at any time in life. It may feel strange to practice skills that others have known since childhood, but nevertheless, learning, imitating, and practicing lead to new abilities that are not much harder to learn late in life than they were in childhood or adolescence.
3. Development is like paddling downstream, driven more easily than other therapeutic processes by the pleasure it naturally brings. Except for shame about immaturity, this learning leads to pleasures and rewards in the form of new freedom, joy, and a sense of agency.

Causes of Arrested Development

While we're talking about development, let's look at how it can be hindered. A family that is overprotective can block their child from gaining experiences in the world. Keeping far away from a traumatic experience or memory can block areas of potential development. Even precocious brilliance and the pursuit of excellence in one area can block other areas of normal development.

Since EMPs are driven by avoidance of a dreaded warning signal/nonconscious emotion, and life brings many types of threats, EMPs often include avoidance of circumstances that otherwise would bring new learning and advance the process of development. When EMPs limit exposure to new information or experiences, new learning can be reduced or prevented in that particular area. An example might be a survivor of sexual abuse. One person might avoid sexuality entirely and lose the opportunity to learn skills that bring confidence and a satisfying sexual life. On the other hand, new learning can also lead to learning that others don't have: another abuse survivor might gain excessive, and not necessarily healthy, experience. That could include learning to trust those who should not be trusted or learning to rely on power and manipulation to compensate for having experienced helplessness. These twists and turns of the developmental process are important in understanding our client's assets and liabilities. As therapists, it is within the scope of our work to help clients make healthy decisions to extend development and, with clarity about risks and with realistic motivation, to try new behaviors and gain new experiences.

A devastating, but all too typical example of avoidance causing developmental arrest is the adolescent who has avoided the emotional risks of engaging with life. This can be a consequence of attention deficit hyperactivity disorder (ADHD) and is often worsened by the easily available comfort of substance use. Getting high often takes the place of engaging in challenging activities. Lack of experience with life prevents practicing as well as coming to acceptance of one's strengths and limitations. Soon, the individual falls behind peers, and shame becomes a deterrent to re-entering the mainstream. Motivation dries up, and the result can be accepting a marginal lifestyle or developing patterns that further increase avoidance and make re-entry unlikely. Another all-too-common result is a life of mental disability due to anxiety and other avoidance-promoting symptoms. For those individuals, finding the courage to restart the developmental process is seriously daunting and will require strong support.

In Chapter 11, we'll look at specific developmental challenges and the kinds of problems that arise when the challenges are not mastered.

The Neurophysiology of New Learning

In Chapter 6, I described how Eric Kandel won the Nobel Prize for demonstrating how the brain encodes information as groups of neurons that tend to fire together. As Pavlov observed, that kind of learning deepens with repetition. It is the same as learning a sport or any activity that takes practice. The underlying mechanism is long-term potentiation, following Donald Hebb's 1949 dictum, "neurons that fire together wire together." What that means is that when nerve cells fire at the same time as other connected neurons, their synapses are adjusted so the neurons are more likely to fire as a group the next time. This process is highly complex (Olsson et al., 2020), but clinically not much more than a matter of identifying new behavior patterns, acknowledging risks and rewards, practicing them, and evaluating the results. The importance of appreciating this form of learning is that it is the kind that builds life skills and adds to the repertoire of response patterns available to survival circuits. That's an essential part of clients becoming ready and able to trade their outdated EMPs for healthier, more satisfactory patterns.

EXTINCTION

The change mechanism called *extinction* was also described by Pavlov but has only recently been understood in neurophysiological detail (Bouton et al., 2020). To sum it up, extinction can prevent a maladaptive response from being put into action. Learning in the cortex sends inhibitory signals to the inner mind, where the outward response is blocked. While that can be beneficial, it has the disadvantage of being temporary and requiring regular reinforcement because extinction doesn't change the warning signal underlying the EMP. Since that warning signal/nonconscious emotion is still calling for an emergency response, the old pattern eventually returns.

When prolonged exposure therapy was first developed, extinction was assumed to be the mechanism behind its success (Foa & McLean, 2016). In that therapy, trauma survivors are repeatedly exposed to stimuli associated with their trauma, but in a safe context where the real danger is no longer present. Eventually, the emotional trauma response will fade. This procedure has been adopted for other learned responses, such as the anxiety that OCD sufferers experience when they refrain from following a ritual. In response-prevention therapy, OCD clients voluntarily (and with great difficulty) expose themselves to intense anxiety, which, with repetition, does tend to fade.

What was not known at the time exposure therapy was first developed was that another change mechanism could also explain the results. That mechanism works by rewriting the schemas permanently, so that the warning signal/nonconscious emotion is no longer generated and the EMP is no longer launched. This more recently elucidated mechanism is *memory reconsolidation* (MR).

Interestingly, the conditions required for both extinction and memory reconsolidation are very similar. Both require activation of the old schemas juxtaposed with new information contradicting the old "truth." Extinction adds learning in the cortex, while in memory reconsolidation, schemas are lastingly changed in the subcortical structures where the old, outdated versions are located. From a clinical standpoint, extinction is temporary and effortful to maintain, while MR, once it takes place, is transformational, that is, lasting with no need for further reinforcement. Since the requirements for both are similar, it is often not clear exactly which one is operative.

This issue with similar requirements was personally important in my own understanding. In an earlier article I published (Smith, 2004), I assumed, and wrote, that the mechanism responsible for transformational change was extinction. I was unaware of a report by Karim Nader (Duvarci & Nader, 2004), describing the distinct and quite different neurophysiology of memory reconsolidation. The transformative change I was describing actually matched the characteristics of memory reconsolidation but not extinction. Years later, when I first heard about memory reconsolidation, I realized I had been wrong. Once again, having formed a working hypothesis sensitized me to new information. Excitedly, I immersed myself in Bruce Ecker's then newly published first edition of *Unlocking the Emotional Brain* (Ecker et al., 2024), and my understanding of psychotherapy took an important new turn.

In the next section and the following two chapters, we will focus on the enduring transformation that has at last been explained by the mechanism of *memory reconsolidation*.

MEMORY RECONSOLIDATION

I think of memory reconsolidation (from here on, MR) as the "Queen of Change Mechanisms" because its transformational effect is rapid, lasting, and does not require periodic reinforcement (Ecker et al., 2024).

Memory reconsolidation takes place when two conditions are met at about the same time. The old implicit learning must be in an active state, while new, disconfirming information must be received that contradicts the original truth, contained in a schema. This causes what neurophysiologists call a prediction error, which triggers the old schema to become volatile and subject to being rewritten. The source of new content is precisely the disconfirming information that caused the volatility. This volatility lasts for about five hours, during which a few repetitions of the new information seem to increase the effect. It has also been found that sleep following the experience tends to reinforce the change.

There is some controversy about whether MR is really taking place in psychotherapy. The reason for doubt is that definitive evidence proving that MR was actually responsible for changing the relevant schemas is difficult to produce in a clinical situation. The standards of proof for such research studies put absolute proof beyond today's technology (Elsey et al., 2018). However, as indicated in the introduction to this book, there are other kinds of evidence. Ecker proposes proof in the form of a logical argument. Since there is no other explanation for rapid, transformative change, whenever such cases can be documented, the mechanism can be presumed to be MR. The original cases on which my 2004 paper was based were exactly that: clinical situations where dissociative amnesia had blocked access to memories until they were strongly re-activated (re-experienced) in therapy in a context of safety. The calm and safe relationship and environment provided the disconfirming experience. Over a few hours, permanent healing took place. Since then, I have seen other pure examples, while Ecker and others have documented many more (Ecker et al., 2024).

Is this evidence good enough to say that MR is evidence-based? That issue is discussed in more depth in the introductory chapter. For our purposes, every official definition of evidence-based leaves room for clinical observation as evidence in situations where scientific proof is lacking. For clinical use, the absence of any other explanation is arguably sufficient proof that MR is, indeed, the Queen of Change Mechanisms. Furthermore, creating the two conditions required for MR predictably results in transformative change. For those who are not fully convinced, I still suggest that the working hypothesis presented here is fully consistent with clinical experience and useful for learning and for practice, not to mention future research.

The mechanism of MR itself is quite simple in clinical practice and makes evolutionary sense. From the point of view of evolution, it serves the important purpose of giving the brain a way to change responses as conditions change. For the therapist, the most challenging part is making sure the two required conditions are fulfilled, and that the new, disconfirming information is delivered to the subcortical structures where schemas are held.

Three Therapeutic Objectives Move the Process Forward

Since there is a good deal of overlap in the requirements for extinction and memory reconsolidation, it turns out that there are just three objectives we need to pursue in doing therapy. They are as follows:

- **New learning builds skills:** As already discussed above, knowledge and practice help clients adapt old skills and build new ones to expand their repertoire of satisfactorily solving problems, including patterns to replace old, outdated solutions embodied in EMPs.
- **Activating the warning signal/nonconscious emotion:** This objective must be achieved both for extinction and memory reconsolidation. The anticipation of feeling the dreaded inner emotion is all it takes to activate the inner mind's warning signal/ nonconscious emotion. Not only that, but simply being reminded of or remembering a threatening circumstance is enough. Regardless of what triggers this neural activation, it is essential to both extinction and memory reconsolidation. The way we know it is present is through the direct bodily responses we identify as affect.
- **Delivering disconfirming information:** This is both the trigger for the two change mechanisms that can modify the expression of EMPs and the source of new content to provide improved responses.

Seeking accurate empathy gives a deep and emotionally engaged understanding that brings client and therapist together as a partnership and leads to fulfillment of the latter two objectives, activating the old pattern and delivering disconfirming information. Those are the topics of the next two chapters.

Key Points

- Mechanisms of change are ways we explain how actions lead to consequences. Common factors are mediators that correlate with success but do not explain it. Three mechanisms are enough to explain the action of all therapies.
- The first mechanism is *new learning*, familiar to all of us, in which we learn cognitively and then practice until a skill is easily available in our repertoire of responses. That is exactly how clients who are lacking a better way to respond can learn and internalize a new one until it is ready to be used.
- The second mechanism, *extinction*, is how repetition of a discomfort-causing experience eventually makes it tolerable. Neuroscience shows that cortical learning leads to inhibition of responses at the level of the inner mind but fails to suppress the warning signal/ nonconscious emotion, so the response is likely to return, and the "cure" is temporary.
- The third mechanism is *memory reconsolidation*, in which exposure to disconfirming information (the ANTIDOTE) triggers volatility

of the implicit learning held in memory that determines how schemas do threat determination and response selection. This leads to enduring change, not requiring multiple repetitions or effort to maintain.

REFERENCES

Bouton, M., Maren, S., & McNally, G. (2020). Behavioral and neurobiological mechanisms of pavlovian and instrumental extinction learning. *Physiological Reviews, 101*(2), 611–681.

Duvarci, S., & Nader, K. (2004). Characterization of fear memory reconsolidation. *The Journal of Neuroscience, 24*, 9269–9275.

Ecker, B., Ticic, R., & Hulley, L. (2024). *Unlocking the emotional brain: Memory reconsolidation and the psychotherapy of transformational change.* Taylor & Francis.

Elsey, J., Van Ast, V., & Kindt, M. (2018). Human memory reconsolidation: A guiding framework and critical review of the evidence. *Psychological Bulletin, 144*, 797–848.

Foa, E., & McLean, C. (2016). The efficacy of exposure therapy for anxiety-related disorders and its underlying mechanisms: The case of OCD and PTSD. *Annual Review of Clinical Psychology, 12*, 1–28.

Olsson, A., Knapska, E., & Lindström, B. (2020). The neural and computational systems of social learning. *Nature Reviews Neuroscience, 21*, 197–212.

Smith, J. (2004). Reexamining psychotherapeutic action through the lens of trauma. *The Journal of the American Academy of Psychoanalysis and Dynamic Psychiatry, 32*(4), 613–631.

CHAPTER 9

Bringing Affect into the Room

We could easily say that affect is the lynchpin of psychotherapy. Science confirms that in-session emotion is a common factor, correlating with therapeutic success. In this chapter, we'll go beyond that correlation to explain how experiencing affect is an important sign that the first requirement for MR has been met. The reasons why affect is so important are fascinating, but the main goal of this chapter is to shed light on how to bring affect into the room.

Affect means all those bodily changes that are indicators of emotion. There are many ways emotion makes itself known: tears, crying out involuntarily, hair standing up, a lump in the throat, change in breathing, fidgeting, heart pounding, etc. Affect is the first part of the inner mind's response. It is first because the mind generates bodily responses faster than it communicates with consciousness. We also know that whenever we see affect, it has to have been triggered by something quite specific, a thought, an image, or some content flashing into the inner mind. It is also likely to be accompanied within milliseconds by some form of automatic thought, conscious content that expresses in a metaphorical way the same warning signal/nonconscious emotion that set off the affect. In addition, the mind's awareness of the body's response adds a dimension to the meaning of the conscious experience. This conscious content may be so fleeting or obscure that we can't quite track what set it off. The usual response, then, is a shrug of the shoulders and letting the emotion pass without knowing quite what triggered it. With mindful attention and help from a therapist witness, the content can usually become clear. We can be sure now that subcortical nerve cells are firing, and that's what fulfills this first requirement of MR. Not only that, but we have a good chance of beginning to discern what events, circumstances, or conscious thoughts may have triggered this activation.

DOI: 10.4324/9781003619659-10

SEEKING ACCURATE EMPATHY

Accurate empathy often grows out of a shared affect. Seeking accurate empathy can be one of the best ways to bring affect into the room. This happens when we allow the conversation to go deep enough to elicit affect, then further widen the channel to and from the inner mind where the relevant schemas reside. When there is a bit of affect or emotionality, it is too easy to lose it and move on. To catch the moment and widen the channel, we need to connect with what triggered that bit of feeling and move the conversation towards that. In social conversation, we might say, "Oh, I'm sorry you feel sad about that." But in therapy, we would want to go further. We might first wait a moment, then say something gentle, "Oh, my…" and wait. That alone says we have noticed. Silence in the room is an unfinished story, asking for more detail. It's time to open our minds to any and all cues about what just happened. Our intuition and curiosity will tell us when it's time to ask a question. Asking too soon will move us away from the affect. The right time will broaden the channel.

As we try to understand the source of emotion, our inner mind and its curiosity are likely to tune in to how this might link to our working hypothesis. Let's not get too intellectual yet. If there are questions to ask, curiosity will help shape them in a way that keeps us close to the affect. It's probably better to keep thoughts about our hypothesis to ourselves a bit longer at this point. After some more time, saying what we are thinking can be helpful by opening an avenue—or unhelpful, as it can distract. Experience and intuition will show the way.

How Intellect Can Literally Turn off Affect

The reason we need to be so careful about turning off affect goes farther than entrenchment and the client's reluctance to face feelings. A physiological switch can flip from feelings to intellect in an instant, and understanding that phenomenon will help with navigating the conversation. Are we in an open, curious, metaphorical mode or a more word-oriented, logical mode? For purposes of accurate empathy and bringing affect into the room, we want to be biased toward the former.

There was a time when there was popular interest in the idea of people being predominantly left-brained or right-brained. That concept has been discredited as a way of characterizing personality, but differences between hemispheres do exist (Caeyenberghs & Leemans, 2014). On the other hand, differences between large-scale brain networks are more revealing than the differences between the hemispheres (Bressler & Menon, 2010). In particular, the central executive network (CEN) is responsible for high-level cognitive functions, that is, attention to intellectually demanding tasks, while the default mode network (DMN) takes care of spontaneous, self-related activity including autobiographical, self-monitoring, and social functions. What is most fascinating as well as significant is that when the CEN is operating, the DMN turns off. That is why digging for memories or intellectualizing about affects or EMPs are turn-offs for the kind of open awareness that leads to complex caring/accurate empathy.

There is another interesting twist to this story. For people with ADHD, the DMN doesn't turn off as readily when the CEN is engaged (Bozhilova et al., 2018). Persistent DMN activity may explain some of the creativity of people with ADHD, as well as their difficulty focusing on attention-requiring tasks when they are boring or lacking in compelling intensity.

Communication Can Get Stuck for Reasons Other than Emotional Ones

If the client seems stuck, the little hint or question or encouragement we might give is the nudge in the three-step dance from Chapter 3. If it helps, that means it was just the right thing to get the conversation flowing. If not, we want to know why. Recalling the three steps in Chapter 3, when the nudge doesn't work, it's time for *metacommunication*, changing the subject to what is going on in the communication. If it's an emotional blockage, then the new subject, the communication problem, is exactly what we should now be exploring. But there are other ways clients can get stuck.

Before we conclude that their being stuck is a form of resistance, it's a good idea to be clear that the problem is not due to a lack of guidance, learning, or practice on the part of the therapist. We don't want to leave the client feeling they have failed when it was our lack of instruction that left them not knowing what to say.

As laid out in Richard Lanes' Levels of Emotional Awareness Scale (Lane et al., 1990), the ability to put an emotional experience into words varies. Some individuals don't use emotion words but can describe what they would do, for example, hit someone or hide. Others may recognize discomfort but not be able to describe a feeling. When young children are told "use your words," they are being taught to use words to express their feelings. In the extreme, the inability to describe feelings is called alexithymia, often associated with psychogenic pain when physical pain becomes a metaphorical equivalent to emotional discomfort. Part of the job of psychotherapy may be helping the client learn to recognize and take an interest in their own feelings. The skill of identifying inner emotions can improve over the course of therapy.

An Example of Seeking Accurate Empathy

Returning to the story of Margaret, she began to tear up when we talked about her attempts to act more assertively and make demands. Inquiring about what she dreaded was what brought up the tears. After a few seconds, I asked about what exactly she was feeling at that moment. As often happens, I could not have guessed the answer that came without hesitation. In fact, if I had guessed wrongly, I would have taken us in an unhelpful direction and lost her engagement as well as the information I wanted.

As described earlier, the surprising answer was that changing her behavior would leave her feeling like she no longer belonged, like she was an outsider. Outsider to what? To the dysfunctional family of her childhood, where her tyrannical, critical, alcoholic father made it clear that she had no right to anything. Despite his abuse, belonging and being accepted were of central importance to her inner child. This was with full knowledge that her father had long since died. Nevertheless, the feeling of missing out, not belonging, was palpable and strong. Her main dread turned out to be exclusion from the family.

That is an example of what accurate empathy means, encouraging the client's deepening self-awareness and allowing our empathy to tune in to the specific dread that has triggered an affect-laden response. The result of that affect and the deepening of accurate empathy is that activation of the old schema, the first requirement for memory reconsolidation, is fulfilled.

WHY IS AFFECT NECESSARY FOR HEALING?

It is remarkable how human it is to avoid strong emotions. We crave them in what we read and watch. They fascinate us when they are being experienced by someone else, but humans are remarkably uncomfortable with their own emotions. Maybe it is because we don't have full control over them, so being carried away is a threat. Or perhaps there are other reasons. People apologize for crying. Is it also because we don't want to drag others into our personal world?

There are probably multiple reasons, but the fact is that humans often tend to skirt around strong emotions, even positive ones. Avoidance of conscious feelings has been studied extensively as emotional avoidance (EA) (Spinhoven et al., 2014). When emotions are painful, it makes intuitive sense that we avoid them. However, what goes on nonconsciously is more fundamental and even more central in the action of psychotherapy. Emotions are at the center of the guidance system for mammalian behavior.

How the Inner Warning System Works

Negative nonconscious emotion is what we have identified as the dread that triggers EMPs. Avoidance of nonconscious emotions is a basic aspect of survival systems (Levy & Schiller, 2020). Once the warning signal/nonconscious emotion has been activated, the goal of the EMP is to silence it or at least lower the volume. As indicated earlier, it works like the thermostat in a home heating system. This automatic and nonconscious avoidance works in parallel with conscious feelings of pain or discomfort and a conscious desire to escape them. Our inner mind is just as prone to seek relief from painful and uncomfortable nonconscious emotions. The fact that the nonconscious and conscious systems work in parallel should not be a surprise, since the use of pain signals as a call for avoidance has been a central feature of the brain's approach to survival since long before the first mammals.

Returning to the role of emotion in therapy, as discussed in the last chapter, MR requires activation of nonconscious emotions in order to set the relevant synapses in the relevant schemas into a volatile state where they are ready for change (Ecker & Vaz, 2022; Schiller et al., 2017). Furthermore, and just as important, the outward bodily manifestation of affect is not only the clinician's indicator that the DREAD has been activated, but also the indicator that a two-way channel has been opened to the subcortical brain. That channel is necessary for the second requirement of MR, the delivery of the disconfirming information or experience necessary for rewriting schemas. Thus, MR requires both activation of the schema *and* an open communication channel for the delivery of disconfirming information and experience.

The transformational healing promised by psychotherapy requires that clients go ahead and encounter their dreaded nonconscious emotions along with their conscious, verbal translations. Neither extinction nor MR can succeed in bringing about healing unless emotions are in an active state. As therapists, we find ourselves in the position of asking our clients to face often painful emotions, hoping and believing that they will feel better afterward. As the wise old German, Stein, said in Joseph Conrad's *Lord Jim*, "In the destructive element immerse yourself."

Is this really necessary? Yes. Now we have a better understanding of why studies keep showing that in-session emotion correlates with therapeutic success. Both extinction and MR require activation of nonconscious emotion. Neurophysiological studies referenced above show that only when schemas are in an active state can the mechanisms of extinction and MR lead to change, and those are the only known ways that existing EMPs can be modified.

Clients often have an additional question. "Do I have to remember?" Let's look at that next.

Do I Have to Remember?

One of the main ways to bring affect into the room is remembering. In doing so, the mind is transported back in time, which can bring with it access to a feeling or experience, almost as if it were happening in the here and now. Unless the intellect suppresses the feeling, remembering activates the affect that accompanied the events when they happened. So, remembering helps activate inner nonconscious emotions, but is it absolutely necessary?

Understandably, clients often don't want to remember because they don't want to experience the painful feelings that will surely accompany their memories. Additionally, the goal of EMPs is to avoid both nonconscious emotions and their conscious versions. It is no surprise, then, that there have been efforts to find a way to feel better without having to experience those painful emotions.

My answer to clients who would rather not have to remember is that they are usually asking the wrong question. "Having to remember" usually means digging for memories. The right question is, "Do I have to feel those painful feelings?" As discussed above, purposeful digging turns on the CEN, which turns off the DMN, needed to make spontaneous connections with the inner mind. Another factor is that digging means trying to overcome the inner mind's reluctance or entrenchment. That runs straight into EMPs designed to keep the conscious mind far from sources of the DREAD. Success in gaining access to troublesome nonconscious emotions comes not from digging but from both the inner and the conscious minds being ready for it. For that reason, more effective methods for accessing affect work by helping create conditions of readiness. Before we discuss that, one more point.

Recently, some "experts" have been claiming to heal trauma without remembering. While emotions can arise out of other sources besides specific recall of an incident, the literature bears out that experiencing affect *is* necessary for healing (Trappler & Newville, 2007). Examples of that might be emotions arising from recurrent abuse over a long period or, more particularly, emotions not from a specific incident but related to it. We see that happening when one learns that a family member knew about abuse and failed to help. Another is shame like Alan's, which can arise from a child's feeling of responsibility for resisting the advances of an adult perpetrator. While specific memories may be avoided, affect can't because it is an essential part of the subcortical healing process. Without affect, the requirements for extinction and MR are not fulfilled. Whatever change might be possible in the absence of affect will be top-down, that is, consciousness trying to impose change without the cooperation of the inner mind. That doesn't work well.

Another strategy for sparing clients the pain of recall is the flash technique (Wong, 2021). It takes advantage of the phenomenon of subliminal awareness, making recall so brief that it does not reach consciousness. Flashing a scary face on a screen can be done so quickly that the inner mind registers it and responds, but without any conscious awareness. This can be used to activate the DREAD without consciousness. In flash therapy, conditions for MR are still met, and enduring change can take place. It may be best for one-time traumas, rather than situations that need to be faced and processed more thoroughly due to their complexity and multiple facets. When fear of emotion is a concern, techniques like Eye Movement Desensitization and Reprocessing (EMDR) can also create a sense of structure and rhythm that lowers the scariness of affect to a level where memories can be faced more easily.

Acknowledging these exceptions, I will leave the emphasis on how we can help clients become ready to experience, then make peace with the affects that arise from terrible events they may have experienced.

MAKING A PLACE FOR AFFECT

We have looked at MR as a neurophysiological phenomenon, but it is also the oldest path to emotional healing, and the first one humans encounter from a very young age. When a child cries and the mother responds with a soft voice and soothing touch, that is MR in action. It may not be the modification of an existing survival circuit, but it can help the child create a new, healthy survival circuit. With consistency in a mother's or caregiver's soothing, initial learning helps the child build resilience with regard to painful feelings. The child's affect is activated, and the mother or caregiver provides confirming information in a natural form that reaches into the inner mind to deliver its reassuring message. In those subcortical structures, information is delivered that this is not the end of the child's world. From that ancient pattern, psychotherapy borrows the essential elements to build experience with new, healthier, and more satisfactory response patterns. The individual develops the skill of sharing affect with a trusted witness and allowing the other's calming perspective to heal the pain.

This is where the relationship-based common factors come into play. Having trust in the therapist and the process is essential. When a therapist takes the role of an emotionally distant technician or when there is an unresolved rupture, the client's lack of feeling safe will usually block access to relevant affects, leaving only discomfort. Then the conditions for MR cannot be fulfilled.

As therapists, how can we establish trust? I have discussed this in quite a few places, but it is essential. Common factors provide an answer. We need to be trustworthy in our words and deeds. We need to avoid making or implying promises we may not be able to keep. We need to respect the client by coming to an agreement about goals. We must be genuine and real. We need to see our client as a valuable human and to respect them as an individual. Simply pursuing accurate empathy goes a long way to fulfilling each of these elements. When it arises from a genuine interest, which is natural for most humans, we can feel confident that we are doing our best to make it safe for the client to experience painful or uncomfortable affects.

Is it enough to establish trust? Often not. Even fulfilling our role to perfection raises questions, especially for clients who have suffered abuse and neglect. How could another human be so constantly empathic? When clients have been betrayed by those who should have cared for them, they naturally and regularly expect anyone, especially a therapist who encourages vulnerability, to betray them. We need to expect this, and when it appears, go through the three-step dance as described in Chapter 3. Repairing ruptures is necessary to clear the way for affect.

Interestingly, it is often us showing our own affect or other involuntary, spontaneous behavior that proves our genuineness and honesty. It can even be the time we lose patience in a way that shows we are truly human. The Boston Change Processes Study Group has identified many of these moments of meaning, when the real person shows through (Duarte et al., 2021).

DIVERSE WAYS TO BRING AFFECT INTO THE ROOM

Essentially, every therapy has its own ways to activate old patterns with their accompanying affects. Here are some:

- **Verbal exploration:** If not too intellectual, asking questions opens the DMN and invites the inner self to be seen and heard. Affect is likely to arise when the goal of exploration is gaining accurate empathy.
- **Transference:** A natural product of any prolonged relationship, transference occurs when old ways of relating tend to impose themselves and create affect-laden interactions. It's what brings inner selves into the open.
- **Voluntary behavior change**: Top-down efforts at voluntary change lead to affectively laden experiences as the inner self reacts to an unfamiliar behavior.
- **Experiential techniques:** The two-chair exercises, for example, are designed to rekindle old, affectively charged ways of interacting.
- **Meditation and mindfulness:** Used clinically, they encourage juxtaposing the inner mind's self-centered feelings and concerns with awareness of an outside context that puts circumstances in a larger perspective.
- **Attention to bodily sensations:** Noticing physical changes can trigger recall or re-experiencing of isolated, frozen affective experiences.

You will find the ways that work best for you and your client. Flexibility and individualization help to make the best matches. Many humans appreciate being seen and treated as unique individuals, while some feel better when they are in more structured, predictable interactions. Our sensitivity to the client's personal characteristics and our knowledge of our own strengths and weaknesses are all helpful. What serves complex caring serves the goals of psychotherapy.

Bringing affect into the room fulfills one part of what is required for MR (and extinction, too). The other part, which needs to take place at about the same time, is a collision between the old "truth" and new, disconfirming information. That is the subject of the next chapter.

Key Points

- Affect is one of two main requirements for memory reconsolidation. It is so because it is our earliest indicator that the inner mind is experiencing or predicting the DREAD, the inner nonconscious emotion that triggers a maladaptive response.
- Seeking accurate empathy is, in itself, a good way to bring affect into the room. We need to be attentive and coax the affect out, with accompanying details, using the three-step dance.

- When clients think we want them to dig intellectually for an answer, it literally turns off the spontaneous DMN. That's why too much analysis too early will block affect.
- When emotion is missing, first remember that clients sometimes don't understand what is expected, nor may they have the skills to put emotions into words.
- Though clients would often prefer to avoid it, healing does require affect. Maybe not a specific memory of events, but the reactivation of affects, indicating a re-awakening of nonconscious emotion.
- Taking time to listen before asking questions allows a channel to the inner mind to widen so we can then learn more.
- Every therapy has ways to bring emotion into the room. Psychodynamic therapies use verbal exploration and transference.
- CBT uses verbal exploration, but the most powerful tool it has is asking clients to change their thinking and behavior. That generates a lot of affect.
- Experiential and third-wave therapies use exposure, role playing, two-chair exercises, repetition, and many other techniques to bring affect into the room.

REFERENCES

Bozhilova, N., Michelini, G., Kuntsi, J., & Asherson, P. (2018). Mind wandering perspective on attention-deficit/hyperactivity disorder. *Neuroscience and Biobehavioral Reviews*, *92*, 464–476.

Bressler, S., & Menon, V. (2010). Large-scale brain networks in cognition: Emerging methods and principles. *Trends in Cognitive Sciences*, *14*, 277–290.

Caeyenberghs, K., & Leemans, A. (2014). Hemispheric lateralization of topological organization in structural brain networks. *Human Brain Mapping*, *35*, 4944–4957.

Duarte, J., Martínez, C., & Tomicic, A. (2021). Sparks of psychotherapeutic change: How therapists understand moments of meetings' contribution to change in psychotherapy. *Psychotherapy Research*, *32*, 511–524.

Ecker, B., & Vaz, A. (2022). Memory reconsolidation and the crisis of mechanism in psychotherapy. *New Ideas in Psychology*, *66*, 100945.

Lane, R., Quinlan, D., Schwartz, G., Walker, P., & Zeitlin, S. (1990). The levels of emotional awareness scale: A cognitive-developmental measure of emotion. *Journal of Personality Assessment*, *55*(1–2), 124–34.

Levy, I., & Schiller, D. (2020). Neural computations of threat. *Trends in Cognitive Sciences*, *25*, 151–171.

Schiller, D., Nader, K., & Lee, J. (2017). An update on memory reconsolidation updating. *Trends in Cognitive Sciences*, *21*, 531–545.

Spinhoven, P., Drost, J., De Rooij, M., Van Hemert, A., & Penninx, B. (2014). A longitudinal study of experiential avoidance in emotional disorders. *Behavior Therapy, 45*(6), 840–850.

Trappler, B., & Newville, H. (2007). Trauma healing via cognitive behavior therapy in chronically hospitalized patients. *Psychiatric Quarterly, 78*, 317–325.

Wong, S. (2021). A model for the flash technique based on working memory and neuroscience research. *Journal of EMDR Practice and Research, 15*, 174–184.

CHAPTER 10

The Art of Disconfirmation

This chapter is about the second requirement for MR. The old pattern needs to be neurologically active, *and*, at about the same time, new, disconfirming information, the ANTIDOTE, must collide with the old, rendering the schemas volatile and ready to be overwritten. The challenge, then, is delivering this new information in the right form to the right places at the right time.

The Art of Speaking to the Inner Mind

Advertisers are great at speaking to the nonconscious inner mind because they know that it is the main source of emotion and motivation. They use color, smiles, relationships, sex, music, movement, beautiful people, exciting places, and humor. All these are ways of speaking to the inner mind to influence the decision to buy. Politicians do it, too, using strong language, slogans, getting the audience to chant, and dazzling them with promises of a hope-filled future. They know that motivation comes from the inner subcortical mind and that reaching into it requires making use of its own nonverbal, associative, metaphorical language.

Are there ways to avoid touching the inner mind? Yes. One place we see contrasting techniques is in televised advertisements for pharmaceuticals in the USA. In contrast to the main message that the drug will make you happy, advertisers are required to describe the dangers and side effects of the drug. They want to do that in a way that avoids the inner mind, so they couch that information in scientific language designed to be filtered out before reaching the subcortical structures of the inner, mind. The same concerns dictate that scientific articles are written without the kinds of linguistic embellishments or rhetoric that

DOI: 10.4324/9781003619659-11

might cause undue emotional influence. The reader is expected to weigh the argument purely on its intellectual value.

What does this say about psychotherapy? We want to communicate with the inner mind, but we also want to protect it from undue influence.

LESSON 1: NO SALES PITCH, ONLY GENUINE HONESTY

We see and receive far too many advertisements and other pitches. Most of us are wary of attempts to influence our minds, especially if they are covert. My definition of manipulation is "bypassing the other person's free will," which implies either sneakiness or some form of leverage. No one likes to be manipulated, even by a trusted therapist, and far less when it comes to our identity, core values, or areas where we feel vulnerable.

One capability far more developed in humans than any other species is the ability to mislead others. We are the masters of deceit, with uncanny abilities to influence each other in ways that are not necessarily what the other person would want. Evolution has made social cohesiveness our main source of protection, but an inevitable side effect has been the equal sophistication of our false communications.

The inner mind is especially tasked with protection against being fooled. Entrenchment, that is, resistance to losing our protections, supercharges wariness, even within a positive therapeutic relationship. Clients are still on guard against undue influence. If we are to succeed in reaching them with disconfirming antidotes, we need to let go of any desire to get inside the client's head without their noticing. Only openness and authenticity will allow us to do so. That's as it should be, since our job is not to manipulate our client into health, but to be a guide and supporter of their own growth. One therapeutic technique is particularly focused on this issue, motivational interviewing.

Motivational interviewing (Miller & Rollnick, 2023) was invented specifically to deal with clients' resistance to influence. Due to the power of addiction and the inner mind's dedication to keeping things the same, reactance—that is, resistance to outside influence—is particularly strong, especially among addicted people who inspired motivational interviewing. The principle is to invite the client to consider different points of view while avoiding *any* application of pressure. In this way, absolute respect for the client's agency is used to avoid triggering resistance.

Reaching Critical Schemas

The targets of the therapeutic antidote are the two types of schemas, threat detection schemas that determine if a response is necessary and response selection schemas that determine which one to select. That means we need to deliver new content to subcortical structures in a form they can process. Those forms are the same kind advertisers use but serve a different purpose. You can imagine what would happen if you approached a client like a salesperson.

The inner mind, then, is always on the lookout for attempts by others to bypass its guards and filters. It is constantly gauging the motivation and authenticity of the other person. In therapy, the client wants to know whether a therapist's motivation is truly in their best interests or guided by some other goal. This takes place on both nonconscious and conscious levels, roughly in parallel. Even if we are totally clean, the client's process of assessment of our trustworthiness is subject to complicating factors.

An important phenomenon in psychotherapy is the problem of misattribution, overlapping with the concept of transference from the psychodynamic orientation. Both mean inaccuracy in guessing what is in the other person's "heart of hearts." We are terrible at guessing others' true intentions because we can't really know them and because our assessments are easily influenced by our own needs and wishes, not to mention past history. This principle appears particularly clearly and regularly in marital therapy (Hrapczynski et al., 2012), where beliefs about the other's motivations generate strong emotions. This is probably the most common cause of marital arguments. "If you really loved me, then you would have…." Both the conscious and inner minds work together to create tests of the other person's intentions, which are regularly based on faulty logic and assumptions, adding up to misattribution.

We therapists can easily be subjects of the same misattribution or negative transference. Our conscious client wants to believe that we are capable, unbiased, and on their side. However, the inner mind is naturally on guard for any sign, true or not, that we might harbor a hidden agenda or misunderstand them. If our client has been subject to manipulation in their early life, we can be confident that they have inside them somewhere a readiness to see the same kind of dishonesty in us. We can think of it as transference, or an inner child valiantly trying to protect against being misused. Furthermore, clients are just as wary of our nonconscious biases as they are of any intentional desire to mislead. They wonder if we are reassuring them because it makes us feel good or because the opinion we express is genuine.

Misattribution Can Cause Too Much Trust

For clients who have experienced neglect or abuse, misattribution should be expected. Some part of the inner self will suspect the therapist's motives to be identical to those of abusive early figures. On the other hand, the same clients, survivors of mistreatment, may also learn to "bleach red flags," meaning they notice the warning signs but have learned to ignore them. That's how trauma bonds are formed, where the survivor becomes attached to someone who repeats the abuse (Casassa et al., 2021). In short, we are dealing with some real complexities as we work to help the inner mind re-evaluate and change some of its most treasured "truths."

What About Our Inevitable Biases?

Clearly, what is required is full authenticity, honesty, and goals exactly aligned with the client's interests and choices. However, this isn't entirely possible. We are all human, and, like it or not, we do have our own conscious and nonconscious motivations and biases. As discussed at the end of Chapter 5, we, too, have inner selves whose agendas can become detached from our conscious intentions. So, what can we do? When there are indications of a mismatch or rupture, here are a few approaches, some better than others:

- **Acceptance:** Recognize when our needs, passions, and wishes are not aligned with the client's and go through the emotional process of accepting that it's their therapy, not ours.
- **Cover up:** Hiding our biases is as dangerous as an unreliable method of birth control. Humans aren't good at hiding nonverbal indications of emotions and wishes, so it's best not to count on dissimulation.
- **Learn about ourselves:** When we are unaware and surprised to learn that we have a bias, that may be the territory of personal therapy and, in any case, time to own our own issues.
- **Informed consent:** Admit to the client what biases we bring and genuinely assure them that they do not need to be influenced by us. This is *somewhat* acceptable and, not infrequently, may be the best we can do.

Despite this, or because of it, honesty, genuine alignment with the client's interests, and openness are important attributes in doing our work. In the client's eyes, we work under bright lights of scrutiny, leaving little room for being anything other than our genuine selves.

Clients differ in their sensitivity and in the degree of their own biases about whether to trust or not. Some are uncanny at detecting misalignment. Vivian Conan, who wrote the book, *Losing the Atmosphere*, about her recovery from dissociative identity disorder, is exquisitely sensitive to biases on my part. She is unwaveringly accurate in sensing interference from my own inner self before it comes to my consciousness. Fortunately, I am generally forgiven for this once I realize and admit that, as usual, she is correct.

LESSON 2: DELIVERY IS NOT GUARANTEED

Let's look at the many ways that antidotes fail to hit the mark to do their work of updating old, outdated "truths."

- A rupture in the alliance has interrupted receptiveness to new ideas.
- Communicating at this level is not familiar to the client.
- The channel isn't open at the moment. The DMN has been turned off, and the CEN is turned on.
- The mode of expression is too cerebral and fails to reach limbic structures.
- The antidote we think of isn't always the best; the client's is probably better.
- The antidote needs to be an experience rather than an idea.
- The client's repertoire of responses does not include any that are more satisfactory than the old pattern.
- The proposed antidote doesn't solve the inner self's existential concern.
- Entrenchment, specific resistance to change, is blocking adoption.

What follows is some detail about each of these issues.

Rupture in the Alliance

When our arrows are missing the bullseye, the first thing to think about is the relationship. Is something going on that is creating a barrier? That's step two in the three-step dance. When resistance intervenes, the subject has changed, and it's time to acknowledge that fact with metacommunication.

Client Lacks Skills

Clients are not always used to thinking and talking about psychological matters. As discussed in Chapter 9, this is a skill that may simply not have been developed. They may need to learn from discussions in sessions and from experience over time.

The Channel Isn't Open

When affect is missing, it usually means defenses are up and the DMN is not active. The question to ask oneself is, "Why?"

The Mode of Expression Is Intellectual

As discussed in Chapter 9, the same turn-off that shuts down access to affects by turning off the DMN also closes the communication channel that allows the disconfirming antidote to reach its target in the inner subcortical mind.

The inner mind is more like an artist or poet. Connotation is king. Using the DMN for communication, the subcortical brain is geared for connotation and metaphor. It looks at a cloud in the sky and sees an animal. Colors can be associated with feelings. Numbers can be associated with colors. Words can contain sounds that add to their meaning. Creativity means putting things together in ways that haven't been done before. These are the specialties of our own and the client's inner mind and the DMN.

If we want to communicate with the inner mind, which we definitely do, we need not only to be authentic, unbiased, and credible, but we need to let our own inner mind participate in the work of finding content our client can relate to. Intuition is far more likely to find the right word than laborious logic. Clients are very different from one another. Some appreciate the language of the street, which they experience as genuine. For others, the same expressions would sound fake and manipulative. The art of relating through images, metaphors, vocabulary, and all the other ways we communicate is critical to making the kind of connection that will encourage our client to let us into their mind's inner circle. That is achieved by letting our own inner mind do much of the work.

And, in case I haven't emphasized it enough, language is not the only medium we possess. Tone of voice, body movements and posture, our dress and manner, the look of the office, the comfort of the seating, all these are ways we communicate. Clients listen to those contents to learn about our inner mind's attitudes and motivations.

One client shared material about which she felt extremely ashamed. She imagined I would be so disgusted that I would "immediately discharge her from treatment." I answered, "Of course I wouldn't do that!"

She revealed a few days later that it was not my words that made her feel safe; it was a tiny involuntary movement on my face that told her my answer was authentic.

Our Antidote Isn't Always the Right One

System 1, "thinking fast," has incredible flexibility, but for an individual client, not all meanings are associated, and their vocabulary of associations may be different. Many associations that we think of may not work in the client's mind.

One remedy is to keep saying things in different ways. A better one is usually to help the client arrive at their own antidote. My experience with this process is that clients need some assistance to understand what the new information needs to disconfirm. Most clients are not used to thinking like their own inner child to discern the deep "truth" that is outdated. On the other hand, once they get the hang of it, their antidote will usually resonate better than one we might supply.

The Antidote Needs to Be an Experience

Frequently, the best antidote is an experience. In the inner mind, experience is information. Maybe the client has had an experience, but the inner mind hasn't yet made the association with the situation in question. It might be the client realizing that under different circumstances, they *have* had the experience of standing up for themselves, or they *have* experienced acceptance and the peace it brings. It may be that the therapy needs to create the experience. One that is universal is the therapist being a calm witness while the client shares a distressing experience. Our lower level of stress creates a new experience to disconfirm the inner sense of danger.

Other experiences come from things the client does. I put a lot of time and energy into helping clients design experiences that will show their inner mind something new. Acting assertively and experiencing that it doesn't lead to disaster is an example. Once an action likely to lead to a disconfirming experience is clear, it may require going through Prochaska and DiClemente's stages of change (Prochaska et al., 2013) to come to the action stage, where the client actually takes the action and experiences the disconfirming results. Here is a list of the six stages:

- Precontemplation
- Contemplation

- Preparation
- Action
- Maintenance
- Relapse

If values are what are standing in the way, "civil disobedience" may be the appropriate disconfirming action. If so, be sure to warn the client about backlash, the wave of shame they will likely experience when they go against their (unhealthy) inner values. In general, we should consider experience as more powerfully communicative than words.

A Better Response Has Not Yet Been Learned

Sometimes the experience is not yet in the client's repertoire. A lack of real experience with an alternative way of coping can mean it is simply not available. When the alternatives are unknown or have never been experienced, who would want to take such a leap? Imagine confronting an authority when you never have? Or imagine how sobriety might look to someone who has never experienced it as an adult? The answer will have to be new learning.

Trying out and practicing a new pattern of behavior may carry emotional and even life risks. This may mean taking the therapist's word that the change will turn out well. Are you sure? In that case, we need to think in terms of informed consent and have a genuine discussion of pros and cons. We can raise a possibility, but we must clarify that the decision is ultimately up to the client. We can't guarantee the results. As always, accurate empathy means appreciating how the process looks both to the conscious self and to the inner self.

The Antidote Doesn't Solve the Inner Self's Existential Concern

What seems like a valid antidote may not work for the inner self. Discussion by Ecker (2024) is helpful for this. Maybe the antidote does not quite match the circumstances or is too general. Even if the inner mind receives it, there may not be a collision because it doesn't precisely disconfirm the old "truth." For example, "Air travel is far safer than going by car" may not work because the DREAD applies to the *possibility* of falling from the sky, no matter how rarely it happens. The answer to worries about uncommon events is usually acceptance of the worst-case scenario as a possibility, albeit an unlikely one. In the case of air travel, that would mean acceptance of the possibility of a crash. Adults can do that, while children, including young inner selves, generally cannot. Transformational change can mean allowing the inner self to grow into the realization that times have changed, and what was once *unthinkable* could actually happen and eventually be accepted.

In another example, Nancy felt intimidated by people in authority at her work. She was expected to take responsibility for actions that violated her ethics. She had decided to leave the company and had full freedom to do so, but she remained afraid to tell the boss. The antidote was not the obvious realization that it would be safe to quit. Rather, it came from recognizing the fact that her boss's angry eyes felt just like those of her rageful father. When she imagined and pictured scenarios where his angry eyes could not hurt her, the fear lost most of its power.

Entrenchment

Now let's turn to those freshly minted EMPs guarding the inner mind's existing survival circuits and schemas. I called them "resistance EMPs." Here, the inner mind sees change as a loss, losing a protection that has stood firmly, guarding against an existential threat. As explained earlier, these new resistance EMPs fit the full definition of all EMPs because they, too, are *entrenched* in the sense that they won't be relinquished easily. They are *maladaptive* because they are blocking the client's access to new responses, and they are *patterns* that can be repeated.

As discussed above in connection with motivational interviewing, think, for example, of people with addictions who are especially resistant to attempts to talk them into sobriety. In those cases, the inner self allies itself with consciousness to mount an impressive array of resistances to being influenced. It is highly creative: "I'm a better driver when I've had a few drinks." "You are into trying to control me, and I'm a free spirit." "I know what's best for me." "You can't even begin to understand what I've been through." "It's my only pleasure in life." "Marijuana gives me access to my creativity." "I use drugs to escape because my partner is always nagging me."

Due to the inner mind's conviction that using the substance is synonymous with survival, people with addictions are among the most resistant to influences from others promoting change. They are particularly reactive, that is, sensitive to a therapist's deviation from strict neutrality and having different goals from the client. What doesn't work is assuming they want to change when they are not ready. As taught in motivational interviewing, therapy needs to follow strictly the client's own motivation and readiness.

In other cases, the entrenchment may be more subtle. The client is consciously on the same side as the therapist, but the inner mind isn't so sure. The rationalizations can be more subtle, and the mistrust may not be overt. Maybe the only indication is that progress seems slow. We need to be alert to subtle sources of resistance. That awareness comes mostly from our own inner mind in the form of intuition, a sense that we are pushing against something and not making headway. At such times, we also need to be ready to ask about the process. "How are we doing?" Checking on the client's sense of things is always a good idea, but especially when our inner mind is detecting some reluctance.

The three-step dance in Chapter 3 is a formula for detecting and responding to this kind of subtle resistance to the process. To repeat, it means first giving a light nudge, and then, when that doesn't work, acknowledging that the resistance is now the subject and seeking accurate empathy through metacommunication. That usually gets things moving again, but if not, we move to step three, recognizing that this subject is too hot and will have to be postponed for another day.

THE CLIENT'S ANTIDOTE IS USUALLY THE BEST

Let's say we are finally in a position to deliver an antidote consisting of clear disconfirming information expressed in a form tuned to the client's own modes of expression. We have done a good job of helping the client access their outdated inner truth in precise terms. One method, demonstrated by Margaret later in this chapter, is writing the old inner "truth" on one side of a spiral-bound notebook and re-reading it as a reminder of the old implicit truth in a way that brings up affect. When that affect is present, that means the channel is open, and it's time to look at the other side of the page for new information to disconfirm the old and generate a prediction error.

As indicated above, what usually works best is for the client to discover their own antidote. What new information can be disconfirming for them? It will often come in a form that you, the therapist, would not have thought of. Carole realized that the sexual abuse she experienced was at an age when the sexual content really didn't mean anything to her. It just hurt physically. In a flash, she had the awareness that her own experience had been no worse than getting hit by a puck in street hockey. It hurt a lot at the time but was soon forgotten. Her lifelong feeling of shame immediately disappeared. From the association with a playground injury, her mind grasped that the shame that had plagued her for decades was her mother's and in no way reflected her own feelings.

The metaphorical connection to a playground mishap put the experience in an entirely new perspective.

Two Kinds of Antidote

I have emphasized the difference between the two stages of inner logic that lead to the outer manifestations of an EMP, the threat detection schema and the response selection schema. One stage measures the dreaded nonconscious emotion to determine whether a response is required, and the second stage determines what the response should be. The antidotes for the two are not the same.

For the threat detection schema, the antidote needs to disconfirm the prediction of danger. The sense of safety in the face of a former sense of danger is rarely limited to words. Rather, it is typically contained nonverbally in circumstances and manners that convey safety and, by implication, deny danger. That can consist of the therapist's tone of voice and soothing attitude, plus the quiet safety of the office. It can also be the client's realization that things are no longer the same and that what was terribly threatening then can now be safely coped with. In the above example, realizing that a playground injury was a more accurate metaphor for the traumatic events was an antidote to the threat of shame.

The other type of antidote is when the selection of the EMP's response pattern needs to be updated. Margaret, who was afraid making demands would result in her being banished, is an example. The antidote needed to be an actual experience. Such an experience could be pulled up from memories or created by taking a new action, in which making demands demonstrably fails to bring banishment. In the latter case, that means overcoming resistance and practicing the new pattern to build confidence. In Margaret's case, what worked was a step-by-step experience in making demands that clearly didn't lead to punishment. For her, these actions were particularly challenging because her stepmother was still alive, still ungrateful, and still unreasonably demanding. Saying no to her was a truly daunting exercise, made even harder because, as anticipated, her stepmother did indeed exhibit shock and anger when her sense of entitlement was not honored. And this was made more painful by the client's residual sense of shame.

A common and important consideration is clients' failure to learn from new, healthy relationships. Margaret's relationship with her husband is based on a healthy give and take, but, perhaps surprisingly, had no value as a disconfirming experience. The reason is that his persona did not create any association between her accepting husband and the entitled people who remind her of her demanding father. As far as the inner mind is concerned, he is in an entirely different category, so his warmth and accepting attitude has no bearing on the old threat. In practice, there are many instances where healthy experience fail to disconfirm unhealthy relational experiences simply because the inner mind holds them in entirely different categories.

Once again, my advice is to go deep into the details of the inner truth and help the client develop their own antidote. When the antidote is clearly effective, then it's time to get out the spiral-bound book and write it down on the right side of the page.

Rewriting Values, Attitudes, Ideals, and Prohibitions

Shame is special because, as described in Chapter 5 in the section on inner critics, it is derived from internalized values. Letting go of shame requires abandoning an unhealthy value, attitude, ideal, or prohibition. The mind holds onto those values with a special intensity because they are meant to help us resist temptation. The process of changing entrenched values is the same as for pathological beliefs, but harder in that internal resistance to change is much more intense. The main factor supporting the maintenance of values is the shame attached to failing to respect them. Margaret's shame about "mistreating" her entitled stepmother was hard to change. The antidote for the threat of shame usually needs to be applied over time with persistence. "Civil disobedience" is creating experiences that show the inner critic how its old value system is outdated. When clients succeed in changing their behavior, it will usually generate an intense and distressing backlash, a wave of shame. The answer to those painful feelings is to recognize where they come from and persist with the new behavior anyway. Eventually, inner critics do seem capable of seeing the light. Sometimes, a specific antidote, as in the case of Margaret, can bring sudden, transformative change.

Margaret continued to be plagued by her inner critic. We needed a way for her to remember that her inner criticism was unfounded. I asked Margaret to use her spiral-bound book to write down the details of her father's scathing view of her, the one that determined a rule never to assert her value or show talents to others. Here is what she wrote:

> *"No matter how good you are or how hard you try, you're not worth so much as a glance up from a newspaper when you walk in the room. Not worth the price of a long, hot shower or a slice of cheese on a fast-food burger. If you think you're smart or funny or pretty...you're wrong. If anyone tells you different, they're either stupid or a liar."*

To avoid her father's punishment and her own internal shame, the rule was this:

> *"Therefore, in order to avoid ridicule, I must keep my mouth shut. In order to avoid anger, I must snap to attention, anticipate every need, please everyone at all times, no matter what. In order for my existence to be tolerated, I must make myself as small and insignificant as possible."*

Here is her statement of the ANTIDOTE. As she wrote it, she could feel its truth:

> *"I don't need to scurry through life apologizing for myself. I'm allowed to take up space in the world...to voice an opinion, make a joke, buy myself something nice.*
>
> *I will listen to the part of me that knows this to be true. And if I falter, I will remind myself that I am no longer a scared little girl. And I will think of my husband who loves me and is neither an idiot nor a liar."*

THE ROLE OF ACCEPTANCE

One of the most common strategies embodied in EMPs is avoidance of having to accept. That's because children are not programmed to accept. They usually have an existential need to maintain hope. Maybe that's because there is so little they can control, or maybe it is built in by evolution. In any case, the result is that many of the best antidotes have to do with the fact that adults can use acceptance to make peace with reality rather than combating it or twisting the perception of reality to fit with their needs. This is how clients get from "that's unthinkable" to "oh well."

Here is a subtlety: An antidote is information that contradicts an outdated rule. Sometimes the contradiction is an idea. "Dying in an airplane is not unthinkable, it is unlikely, but could possibly happen, and that could eventually be accepted." At other times, it is an action whose results contradict the old rule; for example, risking the sight of the boss's angry eyes without experiencing harm could contradict the rule that doing so is too dangerous. Thus, an antidote can be an idea expressed as a word picture, an image, a metaphor, etc. or it can be an experience. Either way, the essence is that it effectively disproves the old rule.

Acceptance is a learned skill. It often comes from painful experiences when reality wins and we lose. In healthy families, children win some battles and lose others. They learn to accept that losing is not so terrible. On the other hand, children who are consistently indulged may never have the experience of losing a battle. It's unthinkable. This can be a source of pathological narcissism. Another source of narcissism is a background of consistent defeat, never winning. That, too, is fertile ground for the development of an inability to acknowledge yet another loss.

Those are extremes of failure to learn the skill of acceptance. For most people, acceptance is in their repertoire, but may be blocked in specific circumstances, especially in relation to threats experienced as existential. Important forms of dread can be powerful enough to block acceptance in specific instances. Examples are helplessness, hopelessness, loss of control, being done to, being alone, being taken by surprise, and, especially, anticipation of running out of resources to cope.

When the skill of acceptance has been learned, the trigger for applying it is realizing that reality doesn't negotiate and that a battle has been lost. When experience with acceptance in relation to a specific dread is lacking, then it may require practice, real or imagined. In such cases, new learning is the mechanism for adding this new area of skill. Accepting failure follows the same pathway as any other voluntary behavior change, but it is often scarier. Role models can be helpful, giving an example to learn from.

Acceptance is a process, and while the realization that the battle has been lost may be instantaneous, there may still be a grieving process. It takes some time to work through the real disappointment of realizing that there is no hope of reversing reality. Grieving is a self-healing process, but must remain on the surface, that is, remain in consciousness, to proceed. Buried grief doesn't evolve over time. It stays fixed. Losses can leave a residual sadness, but clients know when they are done grieving. Then they experience something that feels like closure.

Delivering the right antidote at the right time to the right area in the brain is necessarily challenging. Accurate empathy will lead to getting it right with remarkable and measurable rewards.

The difficulty of delivering disconfirming information to an inner mind dedicated to the status quo brings into focus the intricate balance between the desire to heal and grow versus the inner mind's wish to keep things the same. In the next chapter, we'll examine in detail how motivation is the result of opposing forces and is the main determinant of whether therapeutic change will succeed or fail.

Key Points

- The second requirement for memory reconsolidation (as well as extinction) is the delivery of disconfirming information, the ANTIDOTE.
- Delivering disconfirming information is genuinely challenging. We need to attend to the message being delivered, but just as important is the current state of the communication channel to and from the inner mind.
- Clients are naturally mistrustful of challenges to their inner "truths." If we come on too strongly, the channel will shut. When we recognize that we have biases or personal agendas, it's best to acknowledge them.
- Any unhealed rupture in the alliance will block communication of the ANTIDOTE.
- Given the presence of entrenchment, that is, an inner reluctance to accept change, there are many other factors that can interfere with the delivery of disconfirming information.
- The threat detection schema needs to learn that the circumstances are no longer threatening.
- The response selection schema needs to learn that there is a better way to respond. This is only possible when a better way actually exists in the client's repertoire of responses, newly learned or adapted from the past. Often, these involve becoming ready to accept realities that once were "unthinkable."
- With EMPs involving an inner critic, the change required is to the unhealthy standard by which judgments are being made. These are especially closely guarded and resistant to change.
- The best ANTIDOTES are ones invented by the client.

REFERENCES

Casassa, K., Knight, L., & Mengo, C. (2021). Trauma bonding perspectives from service providers and survivors of sex trafficking: A scoping review. *Trauma, Violence, & Abuse, 23*, 969–984.

Ecker, B. (2024). A proposal for the unification of psychotherapeutic actionunderstood as memory modification processes. *Journal of PsychotherapyIntegration*, 31(2), 291–314.

Hrapczynski, K., Epstein, N., Werlinich, C., & Lataillade, J. (2012). Changes in negative attributions during couple therapy for abusive behavior: relations to changes in satisfaction and behavior. *Journal of marital and family therapy, 38*(Suppl. 1), 117–132.

Miller, W. R., & Rollnick, S. (2023). *Motivational interviewing: Helping people change and grow* (4th ed.). Guilford Press.

Prochaska, J., Norcross, J., & DiClemente, C. (2013). Applying the stages of change. *Psychotherapy in Australia, 19*, 10.

CHAPTER 11

Hope, Motivation, and Development

A therapist asked for help with a client who seemed to be moving away from therapy, disengaging. She was afraid he would drop out. We applied the consultant's first rule: *It's right in front of you, and it's about the relationship.* When we're stuck, that dictum almost always points to the answer, but seeing how may not be obvious. We'll get to the answer soon, but the point of this chapter is that therapy requires motivation, and that's something we need to pay attention to. Motivation is mostly owned by the inner mind, though it is also influenced by consciousness. It includes both the adult client's wish for relief as well as the inner mind's desire to solve problems, but those are counterbalanced by costs. When the costs are too great, or perceived as such, the willingness to continue can fade. Motivation is the energy in the tank, necessary for a successful crossing. Understanding motivation can shed light on the difference between a therapy that works and one that does not.

What Factors Make Motivation Necessary?

Client motivation becomes relevant every time therapy comes at a cost. The following are some of the main costs that can drain motivation. Any of them can represent a greater or smaller deterrent to a client's ongoing investment in therapy. Here, I have mixed conscious and nonconscious concerns because they tend to work in parallel. In the end, the perceived benefit must exceed the perceived cost.

- Time and effort.
- Financial cost.
- Having to reveal things one is ashamed of.
- Conscious and nonconscious fear of change.

DOI: 10.4324/9781003619659-12

- Discomfort of adopting new behaviors.
- Dreaded fears that energize EMPs: There are many, among which are dread of vulnerability, loss of emotional connection, another's coldness and unresponsiveness, loss of control, helplessness, running out of resources, being taken advantage of, being hurt, caught by surprise, and fear of being controlled or dominated.

These factors cover an impressively broad range of issues. Because each one, or the combination of several, can create a strong pull away from therapy, they require a robust level of engagement to keep the balance in favor of continuing.

The SEEKING System

One of the late Dr. Panksepp's most valuable contributions is the way he describes the motivational system or SEEKING system, as he calls it (Panksepp & Biven, 2012). While the biology is complex, two of the most memorable features are that dopamine has a central role in motivation and that the nucleus accumbens is a reward center shown to be stimulated by every substance that shows addictive potential. Of those, perhaps cocaine is the most potent.

What really makes Panksepp's concept helpful is the idea that the SEEKING system can become attached to any goal or objective imaginable, whether short term or very long term, and of whatever nature. It can become set on getting a golf ball into the next hole, becoming President, getting the love we need, or any goal we might light upon. It's what keeps us on the edge of our seats hoping, waiting, and making strenuous efforts.

What is even more interesting is how the system responds to the inner mind's predictions about the likelihood of success. The word for a perceived likelihood is *hope*. We can visualize this as the carrot in front of a recalcitrant donkey and cart. If the carrot is too far, the donkey loses interest. If it's too close, the donkey will reach out, eat it, and go nowhere. When the distance is just right, the donkey pulls the hardest and can move carts with astonishing loads.

Panksepp goes on to describe what happens when the donkey sees little hope of reaching the beckoning carrot. It goes into depression. The motivational system shuts down, and that feels like true depression. Everything slows down and takes on a bleak cast. Hopelessness pervades, and the body slows. This profound and broad response is presumably evolution's way of making sure we save our last ounces of energy in the hope of a miracle.

At the opposite end, when the system is over-energized, we find elation and even manic feelings and behavior. That's what too much cocaine does, causing feelings of omnipotence mixed with paranoia. And to be complete, when the goal is finally reached, the intense pleasure of the chase drops off. Soon, the joy of reaching the goal fades and can lead to a letdown.

Nonetheless, there are ways to keep the game going. After each hole in golf, there is another, then the final score, and then, off in the distance, the club championship. The slot machine might really pay off next time. Think how many billions have been made by dangling carrots at the right distance to get humans to give away their money for something on which their SEEKING system has been tempted to set its sights.

Some goals are determined by genetics and evolution. When we are hungry, our motivational system makes eating a goal. For most people, human connection is intrinsically attractive. Goals can be positive or negative. Multiple goals can compete for which is more pressing. Positive goals involving values, principles, and social and political aims can lead us to accept pain in their pursuit. For humans, pride and shame are especially powerful sources of motivation that, unlike the more intrinsic ones, involve judgment in the light of internalized standards and originate in the cortex. And we should not forget that goals are not always admirable. They can be self-centered, mean, and hurtful.

Addiction is instructive in that genetic factors can play an important role in susceptibility to the attraction of getting high. When compulsion takes over, it can overwhelm the best conscious intentions, demonstrating the power of our inborn motivational system to govern behavior. Using the substance becomes an overriding goal in itself. Addiction's power to trump all other goals, even survival, attests to how the SEEKING system can be co-opted. The only goal with a biological basis strong enough to provide serious competition for an addiction is the need for social connection. Interestingly, fellowship is one of the most potent features of the Alcoholics Anonymous program.

The Specific Goal Matters

For each individual, motivation seems to coalesce particularly around one or a very few central themes. I think of age five as a critical time when lifelong passions are first formed. That's when children first begin to conceive of their lives along an arc of time (Lansdown & Benjamin, 1985). That age corresponds to the time when children fully come to appreciate fairy tales, set in the dimension of time. They start with "once upon a *time*" and end with "they lived happily *ever after*." Within that newly appreciated dimension, time, children's minds begin to incubate a concept of what their life will be about. I believe this conceptualization starts in the inner mind, in nonverbal terms. As it rises to consciousness, it is likely to be in the form of "When I grow up, I want to be a..."

Learning about these life-plan precursors is important because once they are established, they tend to shape choices throughout life. As a therapist, I'm often in the position of working to help clients discover their deepest goals and wishes. These are the wellsprings of the immense power of motivation. In other words, to understand motivation in individual clients, we can think of them as having one or a few central themes that are more meaningful to them than anything else.

With exploration, Barbara revealed her conscious childhood view that she had a right to have the life she hoped for. The context was being the youngest in a highly dysfunctional family where the mother was actively psychotic. Her conclusion was that it was imperative that she successfully manage every problem that came up in order not to miss out on her destiny. That sounded like an eight-year-old. In later adulthood, she became highly competent but not invincible. This became a source of intense anxiety any time she saw the possibility that she might not succeed in solving a life problem, including ones over which she had no control.

These life plans may evolve over time and lead to major life choices. They can also remain frozen, buried, and unchanging, like seeds waiting for water, until they come to life in therapy. When major life plans are ignored, life tends to lack energy and direction.

Adolescence

One of the times in life when coming to understand deep life goals is particularly important is adolescence. As young people begin to break away from dependence on parents and other surrogates, many don't know what deep needs and internal wishes hold their strongest motivation. They may not have learned yet to listen inside for hints and experiences that point toward what is really important to them. Without a sense of their own inner mind's dreams, they may choose a career dictated by parental or cultural values. That can, and not infrequently does, lead to depression, lack of fulfilment and failure. It is critical at this point in life that major choices should line up with inner sources of motivation. In popular culture, this is called following one's passion. It doesn't always turn out to be that easy.

Nancy, a high-functioning mother, has two girls. The older one enrolled in the prestigious college where generations of the family had completed their studies. At the end of her first year, she became depressed and anorexic. The problem turned out to be that the family's allegiance to that college was not hers, nor were the underlying values. It took six months of therapy for her to understand herself well enough to make a choice of a school better suited to her inner self. The problem had been that the family values were very strong, and she had not learned to listen to herself. In early adolescence, disappointing the family by showing her independence represented too much of a danger to her inner mind. She did not dare to stray from her designated role as the eldest child until the mismatch with her inner self was too painful to tolerate. When the crisis erupted, she had no idea what was happening, nor why she was so unhappy. It had to be discovered through talk and self-exploration.

Nancy also has a seventeen-year-old daughter. In their family, every child plays an instrument. However, the 17-year-old began to avoid the hours of daily practice needed to master a difficult musical instrument. At age 14 years, she had freely chosen that instrument, a different one from her siblings. This daughter is much more willing to buck the family's values and chart her own course. She has begun to pursue other interests with gusto and is more than willing to spend hours of self-motivated practice improving skills in her sport.

Her mother is worried about what it means that her daughter seems to want to quit her musical instrument. At 14 years, it was highly valuable for the younger daughter to improve her impulse control and self-management by learning to practice for hours at a time. That was her challenge, and, with Nancy's support, she gained a lot of self-mastery. At 17 years, she is at a different phase of development. She is now at the threshold of late adolescence, where the tasks change. Now it is time to turn toward separating and exploring her own deep values and wishes. Now it's time for Nancy to work with her to learn the skill of exploring her inner values and trying out new experiences to learn about her inner self's sources of energy and motivation.

Many adolescents are not so lucky. For too many, the goal of life from an early age was survival itself. Those are the ones who, when asked about their passion, will answer, "I just want to be left alone." Life has been harsh, and the greatest pleasure is relief. Do they have a passion? Maybe, but it may take time to unearth or even to find it in the first place. Issues of survival will need to be dealt with first.

There are other times throughout adulthood when clients come to a mid-life or late-life crisis, finding themselves without direction. These are often individuals who, for the sake of survival or for other reasons, have ignored their inner life goals. In a remarkable demonstration of the inner mind's capacity to keep track of progress, there is frequently a nonconscious awareness that time is ticking and the chances of reaching the goal are diminishing. This can lead not only to mid-life crises of unhappiness, but also to fateful decisions that can lead to positive outcomes as well as disasters.

In these cases, one job of psychotherapy is to help in the same way as in adolescence, to explore, experiment, and listen inside for the signs of what the inner self holds dear. Is it possible to change such yearnings? In my experience, they are best considered precious individual sources of motivation and better listened to and adapted to than changed.

Returning to the Client Whose Investment in Therapy Was Fading

Let's go back to the consultation described at the beginning of the chapter. The client's engagement was falling away. Understanding what was going on required a better understanding of the specifics. I asked the therapist to tell me more. They had been doing very well for about six months, but now, he wants to reduce to every other week. I asked for more about the client. "He's a person who takes care of everyone, his wife and everyone." That was what I needed. It's not always that easy, but here the answer was, indeed, staring us in the face.

When people focus on doing for others, what they are giving to others is a strong hint about what they, themselves, most want. The client was telling his therapist about the needs that are at the core of his own motivation. Giving to others, vicarious satisfaction, isn't enough. Far from consciousness, the client was hoping to receive the same kind of attention he gives so generously. For the first few months of therapy, his SEEKING system was engaged. The carrot seemed near. Hope was keeping him going. Then something happened. I knew the therapist is naturally generous and giving. Her giving would not likely be the problem. I said, "His intake pipe is clogged." His problem was that he was blocked when it came to receiving what he most wanted.

What his therapist will need to do will require a bit of engineering. She will need to help the client realize that he has a problem *receiving* what he most wants. Gaining hope that his problem can be repaired will provide the pathway for re-energizing his motivation. Helping him see that his difficulty taking in what he most needs is possible will be the key to his re-engagement. In other words, by identifying what happened to the carrot in his therapy, we have the answer of how to bring it back into range.

This newly discovered drag on his therapy is, in fact, an EMP, and an important one. His inner mind is still holding to an outdated truth that he should not depend on anyone but himself. That leaves him constantly yearning but unable to allow his needs to be met. In order to address his loss of motivation, it will be necessary to tackle this newly discovered EMP. In this case, the work needed will not be easy. At the center of his inability to receive is one of those self-critical inner selves, whose fierce opposition to healthy interdependence is founded on an internalized value system.

As discussed earlier, the pathway to healing for him will be a change in values, which are particularly resistant. On the other hand, the drive to recover the warmth and connection that he most values is a central and powerful source of motivation. There is a good chance he will be able to gain hope again of receiving the healthy caring at the center of his inner self's lifelong wishes.

How to Learn About Inner Motivations

Let's look at how to understand the factors that are most energizing to a client, positive and negative. What goals does my client value most? What do they give to others? What are their dreams and ambitions? What are they avoiding? What are they compensating for? What do they want to protect their children from? What career choices have they made? What are they proud of? Where have they been the most successful? What are the challenges at the center of their life struggles? What struggles do they return to but never master? These are some of the things to listen for while we ask ourselves, "What is this person's life really about?" We'll return to this below.

In an initial evaluation, I like to learn as much as I can about the person, their motivations, their blockages, and their strengths before I ask about their background. Later, when I learn more about the environment they came from, it's time to look at their early life. A correct guess, when confirmed, can provide some semi-independent confidence in what I have been thinking, or when my guess is wrong, it can open new, unexpected avenues.

Working with Hope

When we understand the principles of how motivation works and how the inner mind SEEKS what it needs for growth and survival, finding the specific answers is like solving a puzzle. What are the forces in favor of the therapy? What are the forces against it? How can we alter the balance, so the therapy moves forward?

Hope means anticipation of something positive. Future good feeling is the carrot. Much of what we can do to energize a therapy is help the client gain access to hope. The other part of what therapy can do is to remove factors that stand in the way of hope. For the client whose engagement was fading, the key was to help him become aware of how his internal value system saw neediness as bad. That was blocking the hope of receiving, but it could be changed.

Empowerment

Loss of belief in oneself and one's own strengths often undermines hope. At the risk of repeating myself, the best way to help with empowerment is to use accurate empathy to understand the client's strengths. As we reflect them back to the client, they will gain a sense of greater ownership of their own strengths and more confidence in using them to overcome negative factors.

We are all made in similar, understandable ways, but our needs are unique, as are the strategies our inner minds hold to help us with them. Accurate empathy means understanding individual motivations as well as the strategies being used to fulfill them. Every therapy has ways of supporting motivation and hope. Keeping these in mind should be part of our job.

The Downside of Hope

The inner mind tends to hold onto false hope as tightly as real hope. That can block growth and progress in therapy. One strategy of EMPs is to find a false hope to stave off depression and demoralization. When powerful hopes are invested in an ineffective EMP, they can block the inner mind's openness to a new approach. Before discouraging or even attacking a false hope, it is critical to establish the possibility of a new, realistic hope. Otherwise, losing a false hope with no better replacement means sinking into depression.

DEVELOPMENT AND THE DRIVE TO GROW

The role of new learning and general principles of psychological development were discussed in Chapter 8. Here, we look at specific eras of development in relation to the balance between the natural drive to advance versus fears that undermine motivation and block progress.

Anna keeps trying to find love, but it never seems to work out. Her father was misogynistic, impossible to please, and judgmental. From age two or three, she understood that getting his love required being pretty. She found some success with that, but he was always holding the carrot just out of reach. She learned that pretty is everything. In school, that paid off. She was appreciated for being pretty and trying to please. The experience shaped her values and identity. She went on to a career as an actress and married a man as difficult as her father. The relationship didn't last, and subsequent attempts failed as well. With two adult choices, career and partners, she recreated the childhood struggle to please an impossible audience. With those choices came many of the same triumphs and disappointments. Her SEEKING was about getting "Yes" from a stone. Her development had been shaped by her environment and limited by it. In her therapy, the goal was to help her get unstuck in that area so she could trade her goal of trying to please the unappeasable for one of finding satisfaction in give-and-take with healthier people, ones capable of reciprocating in ways her father, ex-husband, and boyfriends could not.

What Factors Form the Central Issue of a Life?

Let's step back from the problems clients bring to psychotherapy and think about people's passions in general. Why does one person put their energy and leisure time into looking good, while the adult interests and values of another person are focused on leading others, and a third seeks to untangle scientific puzzles? Each of these lives seems to have a primary theme. Some are less driven than others and may not have a particular focus other than meeting basic needs. In health, these themes lead to our greatest pleasures as well as disappointments. They are the issues that preoccupy us and that most energize our SEEKING systems. One of those is probably driving you as you read this.

When we look at what drives development, three factors come together. The first is whatever fundamental, existential needs might have been the focus during early life. This might be what primary caregivers valued, or it could be survival itself. In the case of the lowest level EMPs, it is usually something of primordial importance that was difficult to achieve or unreachable. A second factor is the balance of difficulties the individual encounters versus their strengths. These tend to form the central issues in a life. But one more factor has a great deal to say. That is the level of development or maturation at the time or times when formative patterns were learned. To say it more succinctly, both motivation and EMPs are shaped by the person's goals, their strengths, and the impediments that stand in the way. Those factors at each level of development have ongoing impact in the eras to come.

Developmental Challenges Rather than Stages

Rather than thinking in terms of more rigid stages, I find it more flexible to think of development in terms of challenges. Getting stuck with one challenge may not block progress in others. Thus, it is quite possible for an adult with broadly healthy functioning to be stuck in a childlike pattern in one specific area. What follows is a brief introduction to a subject that is well worth pursuing beyond this book: the ways development puts a stamp on the EMPs and the individual styles we encounter in our clients. What I know about development started with an elective in residency with Sibylle Escalona. From there, I developed a lifelong interest and was further influenced by pioneers including Jean Piaget, Freud, Margaret Mahler, R.D. Laing, John Searles, Heinz Kohut, Otto Kernberg, Daniel Stern, and John Bowlby.

What makes development relatively similar between people is that the challenges of life tend to be broadly alike for everyone. But the similarity is somewhat illusory. Each person's experience is unique. Understanding one person may give a starting point for understanding the next, but it won't create accurate empathy. No two people live the same lives.

Here are some examples where developmental issues have left their imprint, in roughly the chronological order in which developing humans encounter their biggest challenges.

- A man couldn't understand why relationships never worked out. He would always find something wrong with the other person and end it. His fear of deep connection and his premature flight were entirely nonverbal and nonconscious, governed by difficulties with **attachment** that typically arise during the first three years of life.
- Another client got into **power struggles** with her professors. She was very bright and couldn't help showing them how stupid they were. Life seemed like a zero-sum game, a choice between capitulating and dominating. Neither worked well in adult life. She had not been able to get past a struggle for control dating back to her second year.
- George, from Chapter 5, sought to be loyal to his father's traditional morals while finding room to grow into a normal, fun-loving adult. The two aims were irreconcilable. His solution was a compromise,

combining both success and humiliating failure. His churchgoing father taught him to be afraid of the fires of hell as his **conscience** first began to form around age three to four.

- A woman seemed driven to show her husband how immoral he was and how he should admit to living a life of moral failure. She was solving her childhood problem of a father who was clearly in the wrong but blamed her. This probably arose a little later than George's issues, as her concerns about **morality** are a bit more sophisticated and less black and white.
- Mary is obsessively perfect in adherence to the rules. She still can't understand why her righteousness doesn't motivate others to do the same. She learned to solve interpersonal problems using the **rules-oriented** strategy of an eight-year-old. It doesn't work in adulthood because it fails to consider complex motivations to do or not do the "right thing."
- Many adolescent and young adult clients struggle with "**adulting**," being tugged forward by the freedom of owning one's life versus clinging to the relative comfort of having others be responsible for one's success or failure.
- Adult trauma can also lead to the emergency solution of holding life frozen in the moment of shock. This is a major cause of adult Post Traumatic Stress Disorder (PTSD). Trauma therapy seeks to go back to that moment to unfreeze the response, so it can take its natural course toward **healing**. This is the specialty of Peter Levine, a trauma therapist and originator of somatic experiencing therapy.

Paddling Downstream

As mentioned briefly in Chapter 8, I'm happy when the goal of therapy is to help a client pick up a thread of development where it was left off years ago. That's because of the principle that it's possible to restart development essentially at any time or age. What it takes is learning by trying new behaviors. Moving on from a developmental arrest brings feelings of elation, just as it does in childhood. It's exciting to gain the freedom of choice and success that come with new growth. Because of those incentives, hope tends to be high, and with it the motivation to do the hard work of trying new behaviors and going through the emotions that go with each new experience.

The main exception to the thrill of growth is shame, the pain of confronting one's immaturity. The value of being a grown-up is instilled in most of us, and that makes it hard to admit to having been stuck in a childlike pattern. Acceptance is the answer, and once past that shame, the going tends to be much more positive.

CLIENTS ARE PART OF SYSTEMS

In most of this book, the focus has been on the individual and their choices, conscious and nonconscious. But those choices are often made in relation to outside realities. There are many circumstances where psychotherapy has no control over what is going on in the client's outside environment, applying pressures that strengthen or undermine motivation. Those can make or break our therapeutic goals. Understanding the client's environment is an important part of accurate empathy. There are times, too, when we may want to intervene with a family or other system (Nichols & Davis, 2021). That is outside the scope of this book but, since systems are often the products of individuals, they tend to involve the same principles discussed here.

Enabling

The most common and unfortunate circumstance where hope can be undermined is outside enabling factors that support pathology. My experience has been that the influence of families can be more powerful than anything a therapist can do. Similarly, when other real-world influences are aligned with a pathological EMP, their power can rule the day.

Enabling takes two forms, a positive form and a negative one. The positive one rewards unhealthy behavior, while the negative one consists of ineffective and harsh outside attempts to control a client's bad behavior. In addictions, for example, supplying the addict with the substance is a positive type of enabling, but nagging can be equally powerful in undermining positive motivation. The positive type of enabling undermines motivation for change. The negative, controlling kind gives the person with a compulsion, a perfect excuse to maintain the behavior. "I drink to escape because your always on my back." This kind of conflict can settle into a "comfortable" status quo. When enabling is ongoing and is beyond a therapist's control, we may have little chance of influencing the client to pursue the benefits of change. Outside forces supporting the status quo, whether from family, social groups, culture, work, government, etc., are all capable of adding their weight in ways that can be more potent than whatever a therapist can contribute. Recognizing this, motivational interviewing gives absolute deference to the client's stage of motivation and readiness.

Working with these forces often feels like an engineering exercise. We are looking at the balance of multiple specific factors, each one exerting an influence on the outcome. The best we can do as therapists is to understand the factors, identify places for intervention, and help our client arrive at informed consent for the choices they make.

Shame

I've seen this once, but it carried a powerful lesson. A mother struggled with addiction. Mothering was highly stressful for her and led repeatedly to relapse. In order to recover from the addiction, she would have had to relinquish custody of her child to focus on her own maturation and recovery. She could not admit failure as a mother and, as a result, could not let go of the child and focus on herself. Ultimately, shame about not being ready for motherhood blocked her own development as well as her ability to function as a mother. She continued to go through a cyclical pattern of trying to mother but failing due to a relapse. I hope the cycle eventually ended.

Forgive me for repeating, but as described in Chapter 8, I have seen so much pain among adolescents and young adults and their families who have failed to launch and are discouraged from rejoining the mainstream by the sheer volume of new learning and growth needed to catch up to peers. The weight of shame at being behind can be extremely disheartening, especially since the young person's idea of what the grown-up version of themselves might look like has remained at an idealized fantasy level. It simply seems too daunting to restart stalled development, especially when substances are available to mask the pain of being left behind. It may take an unusual and highly valued role model to give hope that recovery is possible. Once again, hitting the mark, AA members are urged to share their "experience, strength, and hope" with newer members of the group.

Despair Is a State of Mind

Clients may complain that they have no hope as a way of asking for our help. This is cause for an assessment of danger, but it can also be a complaint that the hard work of change feels too risky. We should not be put off too easily. Evolution has made humans incredibly persistent in living. Thoughts and talk of giving up are easier and far more prevalent than actually doing so.

How can we tell? While I can't give definitive rules, here are some thoughts. I do pay attention to the statistic that says older males are at high risk for completed suicide. In evaluating risk, I like the idea of a *Big No* and a *little no* taken from working with adolescents. The little no is really a yes with an invitation to dialogue, while the Big No, maintained with far more energy, is a real refusal. People give up mainly when they have no hope left. That's why helping clients find some form of hope may be the best prevention against despair.

The Balance of Forces

In this chapter, we have looked at motivational factors critical to the success of any psychotherapy. There are always pros and cons. The ultimate "decider" is primarily the inner mind, the source of motivation. We have seen how the balance is affected by the nature of the EMPs used to solve a problem, as well as the positive advantages of change. We have seen how often the inner mind is swayed by the way a solution is presented and imagined. Speaking the language of the inner mind has the most influence on hope, which can be immensely powerful or nonexistent. We have also seen how outside influences can tip the balance one way or the other. The inner mind's fundamental job is prediction. As we carry an awareness of its inner workings, we need always to be thinking of the balance between hopeful and discouraging factors as they appear to the inner mind.

From here, let's cover our bases by examining what can go wrong in psychotherapy and how to prevent it. That is the subject of Chapter 12, next.

Key Points

- Many factors make psychotherapy an investment of energy, time, vulnerability, and money. These need to be outweighed by motivation, and that is largely based on hope, the expectation of a rewarding result.
- Motivation is primarily owned by the inner mind but strongly influenced by conscious thought.
- Jaak Panksepp describes motivation as the SEEKING system, where we are most motivated when the carrot is at just the right distance ahead. Too far, and we fall into depression. Too near and motivation disappears.
- People have very personal goals, often originating around age five and evolving if conscious, or staying immature and undeveloped if suppressed. These goals are the core of motivation, and we need to be curious about them.

- Often the inner mind has its own plan, and that can affect motivation very powerfully. We need to be very respectful of core motivations.
- Development is using new learning to master a series of challenges outlined in the chapter. When EMPs cause it to be arrested, catching up is exiting but can be inhibited due to shame at being behind.
- Enabling can and does overpower self-motivation. Despair can be a true feeling, or it can be a cry for help.
- We should consider monitoring and supporting motivation as part of our job.

REFERENCES

Lansdown, R., & Benjamin, G. (1985). The development of the concept of death in children aged 5–9 years. *Child: Care, Health and Development, 11*(1), 13–20.

Nichols, M. P., & Davis, S. D. (2021). *Family therapy: Concepts and methods* (12th ed.). Pearson.

Panksepp, J., & Biven, L. (2012). *The archaeology of mind: Neuroevolutionary origins of human emotions* (Norton series on interpersonal neurobiology). W. W. Norton & Company.

CHAPTER 12

Boundaries and Pitfalls

Some of the greatest worries that therapists experience are about boundaries. In this chapter, we'll try to take the mystery out of these issues and help build your confidence in navigating them. The basic reality is that we, as therapists, are here to help our clients trade EMPs for more satisfactory responses. We do that by helping them learn new patterns and get rid of unsatisfactory ones, either by suppressing them temporarily or, hopefully, by rewriting the schemas that identify threats and guide the choice of responses. Along the way, we supply emotional support and pay attention to the motivation needed to get over natural fears and reluctance to embark on change.

What makes this a bit complicated is that the conscious logical self can understand this process, but nonconscious inner selves may have more childlike ideas and plans that come with strong emotions. Not only that, but the therapist's own inner self is involved as well. There is a potential for tension to arise when either of the inner selves, the client's or our own, becomes invested in expectations and plans that can't be fulfilled.

The end points we want to arrive at are where the inner selves join in harmony with conscious selves to make peace with reality, so that the client can live their life aligned with both their nonconscious and conscious hopes and values. As indicated in Chapter 10, when discussing delivering the antidote, two things often get in the way. First, shame can lead to reluctance to reveal the inner selves' goals. The second hurdle is the pain involved with facing the grief and anger that must be traversed on the way to acceptance. Both of those factors can trigger resistance EMPs that work against change.

Our job is to support realistic hopes and bear witness to losses, all the while making it as safe and as easy as possible to bring what has been hidden into the light of day and help our client dare to live differently.

DOI: 10.4324/9781003619659-13

What makes this feasible is experiencing success in the world, as well as the relief and pleasure gained by being in harmony internally and with reality.

Neutrality

The term *neutrality* and the perceived prohibitions that go with it are the cause of some unfortunate anxiety and even therapeutic failures. Coming originally from psychoanalysis, this concept can encourage therapists to take a stance of excessive passivity. In the extreme, it can lead to poker faces, refusal of any real exchange, fear of suggesting behavior change, and general stiffness. None of these is good. Instead, we want to approach the therapeutic exchange with warmth, confidence, and ease. This healthier version is a strong commitment to helping our client along their unique passage to an improved life as they wish to live it.

We can boil the good in neutrality down to one thing: shielding the client from our own covert needs and wishes. As discussed in Chapter 10 (on delivering the antidote), we need to align our wishes with theirs, going through our own process of letting go if needed. When our needs and wishes, usually coming from our own inner self, are not in sync with those of the client, then we must abandon them. If and when we can't let go, we have to disclose our bias. It's that simple. The part that may be the most difficult is acknowledging to ourselves that we have a stake in some goal that is not shared with the client. In addition, there are many times when our goals may be at odds with the client's inner self. That's to be expected, but to deal with those differences, we need the alliance with our adult client. That is the platform that permits facing the whole picture from a stance of honesty. We will need to be sure that our aims and those of the adult client are on the same wavelength. That requires sensitivity as well as thinking of checking in from time to time to be sure.

A Real Example

Carole, an artist in her seventies, realized that deep down she held the "truth" that she was of no real worth and would never have any value in the world. This was the attitude she had experienced as a child, seeing herself through the eyes of her rejecting mother.

In a session, we worked to bring the inner truth to the surface with real affect. As we did so, it was obvious, in the light of reality and in view of the positive regard of her therapist, that her self-critical inner truth was false. She acknowledged this but soon found herself furious with the therapist for a comment along the way: "You've got to help me in this!" I had indeed said it. The words came out as we groped for proof of her value against an inner critic. But what she heard was the autocratic voice of a different therapist, one who was trying to foist his responsibility onto her, ready to blame her for his failure. Her fury soon led to her feeling abandoned and alone. She fell into a deep depression but had enough trust stored up to send me a message. I answered with a phone call.

In the course of the conversation, she was able to connect the depression with her fury and feelings of abandonment. A positive history of my trustworthiness and our successful work together led her to see that she was interpreting my words as if my deep motivations were the same as those of her self-preoccupied mother. I responded that I was thrilled to hear her rage. It was entirely appropriate to the way she had experienced my words. I didn't take it personally but pointed out that consciously experiencing such anger was proof that somewhere inside, a part of herself knew she had value and that her mother had been wrong. That was by far the best antidote to the inner truth that she was of no value. The feeling of depression broke, but we still had work to do in delivering the antidote to where it could do its work. We left the phone call with some confidence that the rupture repair had begun.

In this way, organically and based on three years of productive every-other-week sessions, we were challenging one of her most deep-seated EMPs, A part of her inner self had identified with the aggressor to preserve some kind of relationship with a mother who had been preoccupied with her own professional aspirations and consistently rejecting.

This example illustrates the importance of building a consistent track record of trustworthiness. That helps greatly for the repair of ruptures. At the same time, the example shows how dramatically an inner self can arrive at a conclusion that is not well grounded in reality but based on the survival imperative. This can be a bit frightening, but it is also reassuring that, once brought into the light of consciousness, the misattribution was almost instantly visible as being out of step with our long history of good work.

Preventing Problems

Dealing with boundaries is really about managing expectations. While we need to be clear in the eyes of the conscious, logical client about what we can and cannot do, we must also bear in mind the invisible presence of inner selves with different and often more extensive hopes and plans for us. We need to manage those expectations as well. The main way we do that is through the steady monitoring of our overt commitments and a willingness to own our personal limitations and failures. Above all, within the therapy relationship, we need to consistently prioritize our job ahead of all else except safety and a personal life outside the room.

Dealing with Problems in Therapy

There isn't much we can do about clients' inner expectations until they have an impact on the client's outward thoughts, feelings, and behavior. That is when the inner self makes an appearance, which can be both challenging and promising. It might come in the form of feelings about the therapy or therapist. It can also involve wishes and expectations that put stress on the therapy enterprise. With hopes come feelings, and that is what we have been waiting for. The critical moments are those that have an impact on the client's life or the therapy. At that point, we have a delicate job to do of helping the client come to a truthful, positive, and accepting attitude toward their own inner self while also helping them work out what is realistically possible in the world.

This job is complicated by shame as well as reluctance to face reality, but also by the fact that the therapist, as in the example above, is often seen by the client as a participant, even the cause of what is happening. We need to keep doing our job, even when we may be seen as the source of pain or outrage. When the client is angry, whether rightly or wrongly, we need to remain calm, connected, and curious until enough objectivity is achieved to begin examining what has happened. In the example above, I had no idea what was going on until I received a message alerting me that the client was ready for a conversation.

Someone once asked a fighter pilot how he dealt with panic. His one-word answer was, "experience." I still remember the first time a client was really angry with me. I had the thought, "OK, it's time to tighten my seat belt and go for the ride." Not only is it our job to keep listening, but, as things quiet down, to seek accurate empathy by asking for more detail and clarity. After a few times, it gets easier.

It is hard to keep one's thoughts in focus when this happens, but experience does help. Our first priority is to listen carefully. If the client doesn't articulate clearly what their experience has been, we need to draw it out of them. When we understand thoroughly, it's time to ask ourselves about our own role in what has happened. We don't want to make this about ourselves, but we do need to know our part, so we can acknowledge and apologize if appropriate. Finally, when the feelings have settled, hopefully there is an opportunity to learn together about the client's contribution to what happened and how that relates to the problems we want to change.

It may take a while to sort it all out. Until our understandings match, we still have a rupture, putting further progress in therapy on hold until it's repaired. Fortunately, the act of repairing ruptures is usually identical to resolving an important issue from the client's past. In the example with Carole above, clarifying that her mistrust was about her mother rather than a wish on my part to shirk my duty, her inner mind's rule was changed from mistrust of everyone to a more selective mistrust of her now-deceased mother and others genuinely like her.

When it is the client's misperception that represents an inner truth experienced with strong affect, the first requirement for memory reconsolidation is fulfilled. The old pattern is in an active state. As the client becomes aware of the error, the second requirement is fulfilled, and that is exactly what we are looking for. This is Alexander and French's classic corrective emotional experience. It can only happen once our own contributions have been identified and honestly acknowledged.

Even if our own inner self feels unfairly accused, in communicating feelings, the client has done nothing wrong. Criticism may still be painful, but who doesn't have a bad day in the office once in a while? In fact, when clients do that, they are doing precisely what they are responsible for doing, that is, bringing their thoughts and feelings into the room. Feelings and perceptions don't have a moral valence, only actions. The principle is: *Thoughts, feelings, and impulses only take on moral weight if they are acted upon.*

Here is a subtle point: verbal insults or threats can become a form of aggression. Words can be used for the purpose of communicating or for hurting. As long as words serve the purpose of communicating the client's feelings, thoughts, and impulses, they have no moral implications and should be valued as honest communication, even if expressed in lively terms. Whether words or actions, if the motivation is to hurt, then, as with other harmful actions, they need to be curtailed with enough firmness to stop the trend.

MANAGING EXPECTATIONS

The key to maintaining a successful alliance is managing expectations. That boils down to one very simple principle: *Don't make, imply, or allow to be assumed, promises you may not be able to keep.* One well-meaning therapist told her trauma client, "I'll always be there for you." A month later, her husband was transferred to another city.

Of course, we may not be able to know that our client is imagining promises we haven't made. We can't help that, but when a client's expectations finally come out in the open, the above rule puts us on strong ground. We have not encouraged unrealistic expectations. What that means is that, in the conversation that follows, we have laid the groundwork for being able to speak comfortably and truthfully about what we have and have not done or communicated. In case we do have suspicions of the client harboring expectations that are not realistic, it falls to us to ask and clarify.

Victorian Values

The Victorian era in Western culture casts a long shadow on the practice of psychotherapy, especially in the psychodynamic orientation. During that time, physicians were expected to be authorities, greatly respected and beyond criticism or reproach. Scientifically, they thought of themselves as objective observers and did not consider the possibility that they, themselves, had an impact on what they were observing.

That time was also when high value was placed on mastering one's own baser instincts and on avoiding dependence on others. It was the time when orphanages were governed by the principle of providing excellent hygiene, while strenuously avoiding any attachment between staff and orphans.

Professional psychotherapy was first developed within that culture. The expectation was that minimal communication on the part of the therapist would prevent contamination of the patient's productions. In addition, and perhaps more importantly, by withholding gratification of the patient's wishes, the transference would be further energized and strengthened, and deprivation would lead to greater motivation. In schools, for example, punishment, shaming, and sharp criticism were considered good ways to motivate students toward excellence. Times have changed.

The Revolution of the 1960s

In a massive, worldwide revolt against Victorian values, the theme of the 1960s was to let go and follow instincts and wishes arising from the inner mind. Deprivation was no longer thought of as the best motivator. In its place, encouragement, praise, and positive psychology began to be taught as more highly motivating. These values have been incorporated into some forms of psychotherapy, but the old, Victorian values still make their presence felt and lead to tension within the field.

Culture

Expectations don't happen in a vacuum. They are heavily colored by cultural norms and standards. As members of the health care professions, we are expected to follow community standards of care. But those vary by community, country, and whatever accrediting bodies we might belong to. Those expectations say a lot about our role and what is assumed by clients and professionals. Adherence to standards is a serious matter, having powerful implications for the course of a career. Remaining in alignment with standards may have been simple at a time of relatively homogeneous cultures, but today, heterogeneity is the norm. People are emigrating, and cultures are in transition. This makes it necessary to be aware that expectations and assumptions vary greatly and can be contradictory. That is the reality. Clients have expectations that may not come to light unless we inquire about this potentially sensitive area. Our job is to be aware of the tangle of norms, expectations, and assumptions as they become accessible.

For this reason, discussion of specifics is important in managing expectations, even though it may not come naturally.

Individualistic Versus Community Cultures

One principle central to many developed countries is that Western culture tends to favor independence and individualism. In contrast, there are many areas of the world where culture focuses more on community cohesion. In those places, individual wishes should be sacrificed for the sake of the community. While every culture is different, these poles form a backdrop, shaping expectations toward those in authority and what individuals dare to reveal. While most of the writing and teaching about psychotherapy comes from individualistic cultures, much of the world where psychotherapy is increasingly being adopted is more community-oriented. One result is tension between the traditions of various schools of therapy and the cultures where they are practiced. A major example is the encouragement of clients to talk about their feelings regarding the therapist. This would typically be discouraged in a community-oriented culture, while in the West (and in this book), it is highly valued as a source of clarity and understanding.

BOUNDARIES

At last, it's time to talk specifically about boundaries. If in doubt, follow the rules. That's the best way to begin. Usually, that also means having a clear agreement about what you are promising and what you expect of the client. If there are minor details that won't create trouble if and when they come up, not everything has to be laid out. For example, handling of gifts or touch may not have to be discussed in the first meeting. As long as tactful handling resolves issues at the time, then pages of legal specifications are not necessary. An initial session might end with a simple proposal. "OK, how about meeting next Tuesday at 2:30 pm? We'll continue to work on understanding the problems that brought you in today and how to make things better. After one or two sessions, we'll go over options and come up with a plan. How does that sound?"

From there, my advice on boundaries is to start with cultural and professional expectations, then consider what will work best to get the job done. I have seen how excessive rigidity can lead to an undue emphasis on authority and power. That may be one client's central issue, but for others it is not. Insisting too much on rules tells the client that is what you are interested in. Being mysterious or authoritarian tends to discourage partnership and real dialogue. I have seen how a therapist's practice of minimal communication contributed to a formal atmosphere that discouraged disclosure of the client's feelings about the therapist. The result, in more than one case, has been failure of the therapy.

On the other hand, allowing loose or inconsistent boundaries can also open the door to unrealistic expectations and, just as important, intrusion of the therapist's own inner self, the fourth person in the room. Practicing psychotherapy can, and often is, pleasurable, but the therapist's personal needs must be adequately taken care of outside the therapy relationship. To be specific, significant loneliness or a struggling primary relationship can be a serious liability for a therapist, as they create an inner self that craves closeness. The inner mind is remarkably able to rationalize behaviors that fail the test of "putting our job ahead of all else except safety and the therapist having a life outside the therapy room."

Personal therapy is highly recommended for therapists who find themselves in this situation. A good rule of thumb is that if you feel reluctant to tell a colleague about how you are handling something, you should probably do exactly that.

Support

In the literature of essentially every therapy, there is discussion about giving support to clients. In general, arguments are given for a unitary notion of support, often with warnings about infantilizing the client. For me, the issue is simple. The client is a moving target, a person trying to do hard things to make changes happen, but growing and gaining strengths during the process. When they are struggling and we can offer help, then it is not infantilizing. When they are capable of doing without support, they stand to gain from the experience of finding their way. The relevant question is how able the client is to make the next move, and is there a way I can help that will not do harm? If I can be of support, I am glad to do that. The case of Thomas, the man in Chapter 5, who wanted some tips on living, is an illustration. Possible side effects of support are infantilizing and robbing the client of the sense of agency and satisfaction of doing things on their own. On the other hand, leaving clients struggling when they don't have a chance of success is harsh and cruel. As I have suggested earlier, the idea of enhancing motivation through deprivation is rarely, if ever, effective, at least in the twenty-first century.

In sum, the problem of support is the same as it is for parents. There are times when helping is the right thing to do and times when it is not. Each situation needs to be assessed on its own merits. Therapists are capable of enabling, as well as family members. In instances where there is reason to believe that being supportive is undermining motivation for growth, then that needs to be recognized and discussed with the intention of leading to a change that is understandable to the client. The point I want to leave with is that the subject should not be governed by rules as much as by sensitivity to the motivational forces in play at the moment.

PITFALLS AND WHAT ELSE CAN GO WRONG

Much writing and a lot of research have been directed at ruptures in the therapeutic alliance (Muran, et al., 2021). The bottom line is simple. Don't be defensive but be open to owning your part. First listen, then ask for more detail, and finally try to engage in an honest and clear-eyed investigation of what happened. Your success will depend on the client's investment in the therapy and on the quality of your past participation in the relationship. One more rule: When you sense that you are about to lose a client, go ahead and follow your human intuition. At that point, you have little to lose, and it can be a valuable learning opportunity where humanness might just save the day.

A Few Closing Suggestions

What if your client shows a characteristic that you don't like or find offensive? The answer is simple. Find a way to make that characteristic an issue in the therapy. As you go on to explore it, empathy will take hold, and you will no longer find yourself irritated or offended.

Note that this does not apply to antisocial behavior. At worst, that might require setting a limit and putting the therapy in question.

If you find yourself bored, it means you are not progressing in accurate empathy. Knowing new things about another human is practically never boring. It might be that the client needs to learn how to reveal more or to be less abstract and more concrete. If not that, there is probably an unidentified EMP, yours or theirs, that is standing in the way.

Not infrequently, we find our clients struggling with issues we have not yet resolved in ourselves. If you see yourself engaged with the same emotional issues as your client, you don't have to disclose that fact and may be able to learn from the experience. Personal therapy may be the best answer.

If you are not making progress, remember the consultant's rule: *It's right in front of you, and has to do with the relationship.*

Is the situation dangerous? Is there aggression, a tendency toward self-harm, or danger beyond your ability to contain it? Containment means both participants have confidence that any danger is covered by informed consent and can be handled within the treatment as agreed upon. If there are risks, it means they are understood and accepted by both parties. If this is not the case, the client may need a higher level of care than you alone can provide, and it could be time to acknowledge your limitations and call for outside help.

You are not able to agree on a plan you believe will succeed? Consider bowing out. That is a therapist's prerogative and is far better than agreeing to conditions that won't work. An example is an addicted client who wants their substance use to be off the table. Therapy generates stress and will accelerate the need for the drug, leading to treatment failure.

The client's emotional dysregulation prevents doing the main therapeutic work. If active listening isn't enough, DBT techniques are made for this (Heath et al., 2021).

One final bit of advice. Many errors have been forgiven and learned from. If natural feelings of frustration or irritation come out in spite of your attempts to keep things under control, your loss of decorum may turn out to be the authentic evidence of humanness that allows your client to develop trust in you.

Where Next?

The purpose of this chapter has been to give you, the reader, a sense of confidence that you can handle whatever comes up. Things do come up, and it is always helpful to discuss them with a colleague.

From here, it is time to look at how the principles we have discussed can be applied to the wide variety of therapies being practiced. Essentially, all of them offer unique and useful features. When you understand the infrastructure underlying them, you will be able to add those features to your repertoire and apply them appropriately when and where they will help your client on their voyage.

Key Points

- Boundaries and possible pitfalls cause a lot of stress for therapists. Complicating things further are the various therapies that dictate different ideas about what is acceptable.
- A way to consider the level of support and to deal with neutrality is to acknowledge that infantilizing is possible, but failing to support while the client flounders is no better. In between, there is a right level for maximum growth for each client at each moment.
- Most of the serious problems in psychotherapy come from making, implying, or allowing clients to assume expectations that we may not be able to fulfill. Failure to support informed consent is one of these.
- Culture, family, and local customs provide a background for what is normally expected.
- Feelings only have moral valence when they become actions. Words can count as actions when coming from destructive motivation.
- We have a responsibility to recognize when we can't contain dangerous impulses, including those against ourselves. Then we must require more substantial resources.
- The consultant's rule for problems in psychotherapy is: *It's right in front of you, and it's about the relationship.*
- Suggestions are given for some specific problems that can come up, and how acknowledging our role is key to saving the relationship.

REFERENCES

Heath, N., Midkiff, M., Gerhart, J., & Turow, R. (2021). Group-based DBT skills training modules are linked to independent and additive improvements in emotion regulation in a heterogeneous outpatient sample. *Psychotherapy Research*, *31*, 1001–1011.

Muran, J., Eubanks, C., & Samstag, L. (2021). One more time with less jargon: An introduction to "rupture repair in practice." *Journal of Clinical Psychology*, 77, 361–368.

CHAPTER 13

How This Framework Supports Many Therapies

Having built a framework to explain the actions and infrastructure underlying the many orientations and varieties of psychotherapy, it's time to see how the framework can help support therapies commonly in use. As I have pointed out earlier, it is only recently that we have the basic science to understand the mystery of how psychotherapy actually works. Prior to this century, proponents of existing therapies had no choice but to invent theories that only make sense within their own set of concepts. That has made them incompatible and has been a challenge to the field of psychotherapy integration.

TWO BIG DISAGREEMENTS THAT INHIBIT INTEGRATION

The biggest schism has been between the cognitive-behavioral tradition and the psychodynamic one. Two issues in particular capture much of what makes them incompatible. The psychodynamic tradition is deeply uncomfortable with telling people what to do, while the cognitive-behavioral one is equally reluctant to speculate about what goes on in the nonconscious mind. I'm going to use our framework to challenge both of those ideas, while supporting the positive things each has to offer. If we can get past those two areas of disagreement, bringing different therapies together will be substantially easier.

It's Okay for CBT Therapists to Think about Nonconscious Processes

It is understandable that in the early days of behaviorism, with the desire to establish a new science, speculating about the goings-on in the

DOI: 10.4324/9781003619659-14

nonconscious mind seemed radical and unscientific. Behaviorism was established on the principle that anything beyond observable conscious behavior lay outside the bounds of proper science and should be avoided.

In the meantime, Freud started out in his first, revolutionary cases with dissociated memories of trauma, not available to consciousness. When those memories became conscious with affect, healing simply took place. That led to the idea that unconscious processes were important in the development of problems. At the time, the idea of the unconscious was radical, but it was based on a simple observation that has been made countless times since, that when the unconscious became conscious, healing took place. That same observation was what first led to my interest in change mechanisms.

As time went on, psychodynamic therapists and thinkers went far beyond traumatic memories to build effective treatment based on making sense of nonconscious motivations as well as clashes between incompatible nonconscious desires, which they termed *intrapsychic conflicts*. Every interpretation was an experiment, giving a chance for the therapist to observe whether their understanding helped or hindered progress. With 130 years of continuous experience on every continent, it is not a good bet to assume that all this observation and analysis is imaginary and not to be taken seriously.

Approaching the issue from the ground up, our framework comes from a different point of view, one that can make sense within both the CBT and the psychodynamic orientations. We are looking at nonconscious information processing and emotions as an essential and basic part of evolution's design for survival in a complex and changing environment. That is no longer radical. Just as evolutionary biologists hold theories about selective advantage in areas where proof is not possible, we recognize that our knowledge about nonconscious mental operations is indirect and often cannot be proven directly. What we have is evidence based on observing feelings of "resonance" and on the clinical consequences of interventions based on our theories. This kind of evidence is familiar and non-controversial within the psychodynamic realm. In the world of CBT, formulation, that is theories about causation, are increasingly popular. Here it is proposed that, with acknowledgment of doubt, there is a great deal to be gained by using our understanding of the inner mind's processes to make sense of the purposefulness of nonconscious products that behaviorists talk about every day: core values, core beliefs, and the automatic thoughts, spontaneous emotions, and impulses that reflect them.

So, let's join with Kwon and Silva (2020) and invite our CBT colleagues to go ahead and form working hypotheses about what's going on behind the scenes in the inner mind to help with navigating the therapeutic space.

It's Okay for PDT Therapists to Tell Clients What to Do

This argument is very similar to the one above in questioning an old taboo that has faded but still casts a significant shadow. In our framework, voluntary changes in behavior have two very important roles in psychotherapy. The first is that through them, clients can try out and practice new response patterns that can then become part of their repertoire of available responses. We have argued that there must be an improved response available if our clients are to trade their EMPs for better responses. We can leave clients to figure this out for themselves, but when we have experience and knowledge, why not help them be aware of alternatives and provide a place to discuss the pros, cons, and dangers of trying something new?

The second role of voluntary behavior change is every bit as important as the first. Action leads to experience, and experience is one of the most compelling and important sources of nonverbal information. It is a form of information that is naturally delivered to the inner, nonconscious mind. I'll go further. Even voluntary changes in thinking, the kind that are constantly proposed in CBT therapy, can also create experiences and communicate with the inner mind. Thus, telling people what to do and even helping them adopt new ways to think both make sense within the context of psychodynamically oriented therapy.

Carole dared to try out owning her power with her domineering husband. In the days after, she had massive waves of shame and self-criticism. The experience carried a message that shook her existing core value that she should never exercise any power whatsoever. We worked through the shame and how it was, in itself, part of an EMP designed in childhood to keep her safe. After that, she began to experiment with holding her own in the marriage. The balance between partners shifted for the better, and now she feels more equal and freer to insist on fairness between them. Her husband still objects, but, if anything, less strenuously than before. Meanwhile, her inner mind's prediction of disaster has not happened.

There are good reasons why helping people with what to do can be productive. What about reasons against doing so? Just as behaviorists have held a kind of taboo against speculating about the nonconscious mind, psychodynamic thinkers have argued against telling people what to do. It will infantilize them and take away the satisfaction of figuring things out for themselves. Yes, that is possible, but, as I have said several times, leaving clients floundering when we have helpful knowledge is not therapeutic. There are genuine dangers from giving bad advice or allowing a client's inner self to use our suggestions to make us responsible for their failures. Those are real, and we do need to be careful in the way we propose an action or a thought. We need to take into account the possibility that it can be taken as an order, misunderstood, or used by a client to avoid listening to their own self and ideas.

There is one more argument. The earliest one raised against being an active therapist was that our engagement would drown out the subtleties of the transference. My experience is that the will and plans of inner selves are exceedingly powerful and readily impose themselves in spite of our level of activity as therapists. This is especially true if we show an interest and respect for inner selves and the plans they bring to the party.

On balance, a blanket prohibition against suggesting or discussing voluntary behavior change will be more of a drag on therapeutic results than the risk of our ideas or suggestions doing harm, particularly when we observe appropriate precautions. Much of the time, the most effective path is a willingness to participate in discussions of how to improve behavior and thinking, while making sure we don't do harm by becoming trapped by our words or by making the therapy our therapy instead of the client's.

Incompatibilities

These two issues cover the majority of incompatibilities that make adherents of one orientation say not to mix their techniques with those from another orientation. In contrast to taboos, a better answer is to be thoughtful about the safety concerns that go with being an active therapist and with having working hypotheses. Those caveats and the concerns outlined in Chapter 12 give us a sense of what we need in order to protect our clients and ourselves against the harm that is still possible with something as powerful as psychotherapy.

Next, let's apply the methodology suggested earlier of looking for the three clinical objectives embedded in diverse therapies. We'll start with CBT and PDT.

INTEGRATING CBT AND PDT

How can we bring diverse therapies under one roof so we can benefit from the good in all of them? The simple answer is to look at the three clinical objectives discussed in Chapter 8 that allow all therapies to work:

1. Support new learning to internalize improved response patterns.
2. Activate unconscious emotion so as to bring relevant affects into the room.
3. Discover antidotes that are effective in disconfirming outdated schemas and deliver them to the inner mind on its terms.

Those are the essential objectives that lead directly to positive change, no matter what set of techniques we might be using. Since we know what we want to happen, we don't have to be so pure about the source of the most effective technique for a given client or circumstance. We can and should also consider the therapist's own knowledge and experience. Furthermore, as we understand how each therapy incorporates those three clinical objectives, we can see how therapies are fundamentally the same. With our framework, we have the equivalent of a Rosetta Stone to translate from one to the other. So, let's analyze each of several therapies according to how each one fulfills the three objectives.

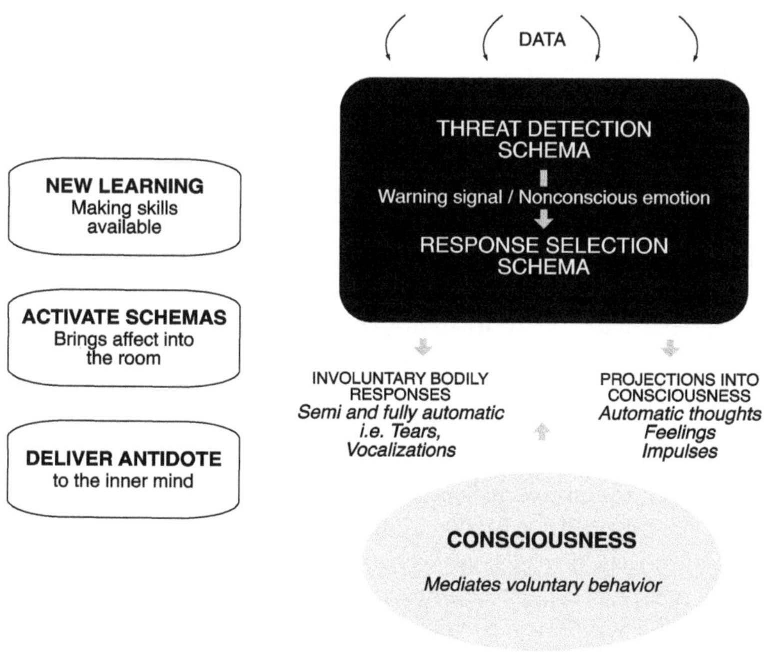

Figure 13.1 Three Clinical Objectives

Cognitive-Behavioral Therapy

New learning: This is an overt and important objective in CBT, so we don't have to look far to see how therapists assign homework and discuss ways to change behavior that will make life better. CBT also incorporates ways to protect against bad suggestions and the misuse of good ones.

Affect in the room: Judith Beck (2021) considers emotions to be of primary importance to the cognitive therapist. She explains that the goal is to listen, acknowledge, and calm down most negative emotions. The suggested process for lowering the volume of a painful emotion is exactly what our framework suggests: to respond with a calming attitude and larger perspective. From our vantage point, we hope, as learned from exposure therapy, that the therapist allows even painful affects to be fully experienced before turning to disconfirmation, known in CBT circles as cognitive restructuring.

Our framework might also suggest a higher level of interest and curiosity about the specific origins of an affect. We see those affects (except for the instrumental and defensive emotions described in Chapter 3) as responses to the inner mind's dread, and we are avidly interested in deepening our understanding of their origin and purpose so we can be more specific in helping clients find better solutions.

By supporting voluntary changes in behavior and thinking, CBT also acts to create surprising new experiences, which generate affects and conscious feelings. Once again, as in the case of Carole above, we are particularly interested in understanding the emotional impact of those new ways of behaving and thinking.

Finding antidotes: CBT is constantly concerned with formulating the right disconfirming information to accomplish cognitive restructuring. That fits with our framework. CBT seeks to craft antidotes that are close enough to the client's issue to shed light on a problematic core belief. At the same time, antidotes must precisely match the client's concern, as we have discussed in Chapter 10.

Delivery to the inner mind: As discussed above, CBT may not conceptualize the nonverbal informational content embodied in a calm presence or soothing language and metaphors. These are nonetheless built into the practice of working with emotions. In addition, as CBT therapists strive for cognitive restructuring, they are necessarily aware that the way a new idea or perspective is expressed can impact its effectiveness.

What we might suggest, based on our framework, is that more thought be given to the juxtaposition in time of affect entering the room with suggestions of new ways to see things expressed in terms designed to reach the inner mind. They need to take place at about the same time for success with memory reconsolidation. When this is not the case, the remaining mechanism is extinction, which, as has been repeated, has the disadvantage of being temporary.

By accomplishing all three of the main objectives, CBT is compatible with the framework we have built.

Psychodynamic Psychotherapy (PDT)

New learning: PDT (Gabbard, 2017) tends to be reluctant to initiate new learning, but recognizes its value when clients report that they are trying out something new. This behavior change is thought of as part of working through and is done with habit patterns following transformative change. As indicated above, we might suggest that a more active stance favoring positive changes in behavior, if taken carefully, can further enhance results.

Affect in the room: PDT is well attuned to affect coming into the room and incorporates a strong interest in understanding why affect is present and what it tells about inner processes.

Finding antidotes: PDT recognizes interpretations as the main delivery route for what we call antidotes. In addition, much modern thinking recognizes the important messaging that comes from events in the relationship and from moments of meeting, where unplanned human interactions can carry important meaning.

Delivery to the inner mind: PDT generally understands the art and the importance of communicating in modes that are native to the inner mind. We might suggest that affect should be used as a marker for the timing of interpretations as an indicator that there is an open channel with the inner self. Timing interpretation and new insight according to the presence of affect is needed to fulfill the requirements for transformative change by memory reconsolidation.

ADDITIONAL CONTEMPORARY THERAPIES

Dialectical Behavior Therapy

DBT is specialized for clients who have trouble managing their emotions and impulsive behavior, often called states of dysregulation. The dialectical part means going back and forth between empathic listening to help calm the fires, then teaching techniques for managing stressful and triggering situations. A good starting place is Marsha Linehan's DBT Skills Training Manual, 2 Ed (2015).

New learning: DBT embraces new learning with a strong emphasis on skills and a valuable repertoire of them designed for managing emotions, each one with an acronym to make them readily accessible to clients when needed.

Affect in the room: This is one of those situations where affect is already in the room, in excess, so that no special techniques are needed. The exception is when action is used as a substitute for feeling. Then, managing acting-out behaviors is the appropriate route used to bringing affect into the room. DBT receives kudos for handling this kind of affect.

Finding antidotes: Once dysregulation is under control, DBT reverts to its parent treatment CBT, for approaches to cognitive restructuring, which are compatible with our framework, especially when attention is paid to the details and sources of automatic thoughts, core beliefs, and core values.

Delivery to the inner mind: The inner mind is heavily involved as the indirect author of dysregulated emotional and behavioral responses. Strong affects mean a communication channel is open from the beginning. The empathic side of the dialectic is directly aimed at communicating with the inner mind in a calming way, while the recommended client skills are designed to give a feeling of empowerment for clients to manage their own emotions. That support of personal agency is a communication to the inner mind as well. Overall, DBT incorporates strong measures to support the delivery of communications to the inner mind.

Existential Therapy

This form of talk therapy emphasizes acknowledgment of mortality and the limitations of human life, as well as freedom of choice. The therapy encourages a mature awareness of the human condition, including the fact that we are ultimately alone, that meaning is what we make of it, and that we have the freedom and responsibility to shape our lives. A strong proponent is Irvin Yalom, whose book, *The Gift of Therapy: An Open Letter to a New Generation of Therapists and their Patients* (2009), is an excellent resource for any therapist.

New learning: Clients are encouraged to chart their own course in life. Doing so often means adopting a more mature, accepting, and philosophical stance in place of the immature and frozen attitudes embodied in EMPs. This implies a strong role for learning new skills and patterns of the client's own invention. In that way, existential therapy strongly supports new learning.

Affect in the room: Existential therapy supports bringing affect into the room through its emphasis on relinquishing comfortable illusions and accepting reality on its terms. Letting go of comforting but "dishonest" EMPs will automatically bring affect into the room, especially as the therapy challenges entrenched patterns.

Finding antidotes: Clients are encouraged and expected to find their own antidotes to EMPs. The emphasis is on recognizing what illusions need to be let go and what realities need to be accepted on their terms. This supports the disconfirmation of old patterns. The therapist's modeling of acceptance of reality on its terms is a powerful antidote for many EMPs.

Delivery to the inner mind: The emphasis on full honesty and acknowledgment of reality can be expected to open the channel to the inner mind as long as excessive intellectualization is avoided.

Prolonged Exposure Therapy

This technique, introduced originally by Edna Foa (Foa et al., 2007), is profoundly intertwined with the mechanism of *extinction*, used originally to explain therapeutic results. Trauma clients, as well as others whose EMPs involve avoidance of troublesome experiences, are asked to undergo gradual exposure to their worst anxieties and fears in a controlled environment, without using methods to soften the experience. The expectation, in line with Pavlov's findings, is that with repeated exposure, the emotional response will diminish. We have discussed the differences between exposure and memory reconsolidation, where MR requires fewer repetitions and can have more lasting results (Vaverková et al., 2020). In clinical practice, it is often not clear which of the two mechanisms is responsible for a reduction in the reaction to a troubling memory.

New learning: This is central to exposure therapy in that clients are encouraged to learn from experience that facing their anxiety and discomfort gives better relief than EMPs designed to avoid such experiences. They also gain a sense of agency and control, where the ineffectiveness of their EMP's strategies for managing anxiety actually tends to increase the sense of being at the mercy of circumstances.

Affect in the room: Central to this therapy, affect is purposefully generated by exposure, whether in imagination or through tangible reminders. Techniques are calculated to maximize the experience of strong affect to the extent that it can be tolerated.

Finding antidotes: A lowering of distress with painful memories provides experiential antidotes to the client's dread of recall. Furthermore, the safety of the setting and calm of the therapist are, in themselves, disconfirming of the inner mind's perception of danger.

Delivery to the inner mind: As an experiential technique, conducted with full affect in the room, the channel is wide open for communication with the inner self. The exception may be that multiple repetitions of a painful memory may be counterproductive by biasing towards extinction rather than memory reconsolidation.

Acceptance and Commitment Therapy

The principles of ACT start with acceptance, mindfulness, and the observing self (Hayes, 2016). I admire Steven Hayes, the originator of ACT, as someone who has looked deeper into the workings of psychotherapy than many. He is one behaviorally oriented therapist who identifies survival circuits as nonconscious sources of the problems psychotherapy treats (Hayes & Hofmann, 2018).

New learning: The commitment part of ACT is where clients commit to adopting new patterns of response. In doing this, it embraces the need for new response patterns. These new patterns not only improve satisfaction in life but also provide disconfirming experiential content to collide with outdated "truths."

Affect in the room: The suggestion that acceptance is helpful is automatically challenging to EMPs that include emotional avoidance (EA) as a means of avoiding acceptance. Consistent with its roots in the behavioral tradition (this is one of the "third wave" behavioral treatments), the concept of EA focuses on conscious experience and doesn't mention nonconscious emotion. Nonetheless, a primary goal of ACT is to encourage the experience of emotion. In our framework, avoidance of nonconscious emotion is a fundamental feature of EMPs, and a central element in making sense of both nonconscious and conscious patterns of avoidance.

Finding antidotes: This therapy recognizes that when the inner mind is frozen in time, the client loses sight of an outside perspective. The concept of cognitive defusion means helping clients go beyond the state where subjective experience is taken as reality and looking mindfully at painful experiences as a mental phenomenon. The commitment part of the therapy places strong emphasis on learning and practicing improved response patterns, which provide experiential antidotes to contradict the inner mind's expectations.

Delivery to the inner mind: As a deeply experiential therapy, ACT takes advantage of nonverbal communication channels with the inner mind that open in the presence of affect and receive disconfirming information in the form of experience.

Emotion Focused Therapy

Emotion focused therapy (Greenberg, 2006) focuses on interpersonal relationships and the strong emotions evoked within them. Discussion of outside relationships is combined with a context where the therapeutic relationship is central. These are both sources of corrective emotional experiences, in which affect is generated by the inquiry and juxtaposed with corrective experience within the relational bond. What that means is that, as described in Chapter 7, "emotion is healed with emotion." The experience of a new, benign emotion provides disconfirmation of the old schemas and their dreaded negative affects. The approach emphasizes circular psychodynamics in which EMPs are triggered in relationships, which then lead to maladaptive responses from the other person, embedded in repeating cycles. Clients stuck in these cycles learn healthier ways of responding (new learning) and incorporate them in their lives.

Homework is different in emphasis from CBT in that it tends to focus on practicing awareness of emotions and patterns of response in relation to other people and the environment, in contrast to cognitive restructuring.

New learning: Trying out new responses is central to EFT, with emphasis on learning from the therapist's modeling and from the client's practicing new ways of responding to triggering circumstances, especially in the context of relationship patterns.

Affect in the room: Experiencing affect is central in EFT. It is encouraged by the focus on observing and exploring patterns of interaction that trigger emotions and the experience of emotions themselves. Accurate empathy is a natural result of this therapy.

Finding antidotes: This is where "healing emotion with emotion" represents using new emotional experiences as antidotes to old, self-absorbed emotional experiences. In this way, the therapy is experiential, implying that it favors this powerful form of nonverbal disconfirming information, especially as it pertains to EMPs that involve relationships.

Delivery to the inner mind: The central role of affect leads to a strong emphasis on conditions that create and maintain an open channel with the inner mind as well as the use of experience, which then has native access to the inner mind.

Eye Movement Desensitization and Reprocessing

Eye Movement Desensitization and Reprocessing, EMDR (Leeds, 2016) is mainly aimed at trauma. Periods of free association in relation to troubling memories alternate with times of quiet while experiencing alternating stimuli. This structure provides soothing boundaries and a regular rhythm. The exact function of bilateral stimuli, such as clicking sounds, is still a matter of debate, but they seem to distract the intellect and facilitate the opening of channels for two-way communication with the inner mind. The aim, as in exposure therapy, is to lower the subjective distress associated with painful experiences and circumstances, but repetition is not forced. Rather, the therapy encourages the spontaneous sharing of whatever content comes to mind.

New learning: New learning of alternative response patterns is called the "installation" of more adaptive truths and responses. Here, the client focuses on the new pattern, then experiences alternating stimuli to facilitate communication into the inner mind. The experience of mastery is also learned as an alternative to feeling at the mercy of painful memories.

Affect in the room: The procedure emphasizes openness to spontaneous material from within, which leads to affective awareness and tolerance of emotions around what is dreaded.

Finding antidotes: Note that in trauma, the emphasis is on changing the threat detection schema, so it no longer registers a threat. In such cases, the context of safety and calm is the antidote, communicated experientially to the inner mind. This sense of calm combines the soothing structure of the procedure with the accurate empathy that arises from the client's sharing free associations to the distressing material.

Delivery to the inner mind: The emphasis on spontaneous free association and on accessing affectively charged material is effective in keeping open the communication channel to and from the inner mind.

IFS, Internal Family Systems Therapy

This therapy (Brenner, 2023) differentiates inner selves into *managers*, who work to keep dreaded nonconscious emotions under control, while *firefighters* deal with emergencies and the threat of dysregulation. By entering into personified dialog with these parts, the therapist and client can establish accurate empathy and help each part work out the threats and EMP responses it has adopted for protection. These parts are the same as the inner selves referred to in this book.

In addition to the conscious, here-and-now client and the inner protectors, the therapy also identifies a deeper inner "self" who is aware of reality and knows what is needed. We got a glimpse of that self in Chapter 12, when Carole realized that a part of her already knew that she had value. That self was present somewhere behind the scenes.

Each of the parts identified in IFS engages in therapy by doing the same things we have seen in other therapies, learning new patterns, activating outdated responses, and taking in disconfirming points of view, such that old schemas can be rewritten. The difference is that the dialog can be directly engaged with an often-childlike inner self. One of the classic interventions of IFS is, "What would it be like if you didn't have to...?" The rest of the sentence encourages the part to reflect on what it does to keep everything under control. This capitalizes on the part's exhaustion as it toils to ensure safety. The wish to take a rest is used as motivation for change. It also makes use of surprise to encourage a reflective state. It's an excellent way to deliver disconfirming information to shake up an old "truth."

New learning: IFS is basically experiential, encouraging changes in outdated protective patterns.

Affect in the room: Inner selves are lively sources of real-time affect. Contacting them in their own "frozen in time" environment strongly encourages contact with affect.

Finding antidotes: These are generally experiential as a result of introducing new ways of looking at behaviors and ways of understanding life that have been taken for granted and assumed to be the only possible versions of reality.

Delivery to the inner mind: Contact with inner selves automatically opens a strong two-way communication channel established in direct dialogue with the inner self.

USING OUR ROSETTA STONE

I hope it is clear by this time that these therapies and untold others make use of the same three clinical objectives and three change mechanisms at the center of this book. Within our framework, the goal of seeking accurate empathy provides a single focus that is useful in promoting each of the three objectives

In every therapy, there are paths for recognizing, activating, and understanding EMPs, while experiencing their associated affects. From there, psychotherapy provides many pathways for delivering new, disconfirming information and adopting healthier responses. What makes therapies distinct is that each has a different style and appeal, both for therapists and clients.

With an outline for understanding the features that underlie essentially all of them, we can understand why no one approach is better than all the others. They all fulfill the same objectives and make use of the same change processes. That is reassuring, but more importantly, knowing what is going on underneath leads us to see more clearly how to match techniques to the individual client and to what is needed in the moment.

Psychotherapy Integration

My first exposure to the mixing of techniques from different therapies was in residency. Helen Singer Kaplan, a pioneer in her field, gave a lecture on sex therapy. She explained how the technique involved giving behavioral homework, which couples routinely failed to do. Then, she described using psychodynamic techniques to help the couple explore the meaning of why they didn't do the homework. From there, they would learn about maladaptive patterns and their source, fulfilling the three objectives that are part of every psychotherapy.

Some years later, when Rob Feinstein, my training director, asked me to teach a class on mixing psychodynamic and cognitive-behavioral techniques, I immediately accepted because that is what I had been doing for some time. That assignment was what led me to the Society for the Exploration of Psychotherapy Integration.

The relevance to this book is that when we know the benefits and possible side effects of the things we do, we can see in advance how different techniques can or cannot be mixed. For example, when working with Margaret, we first explored the dread she experienced simply by thinking of a new behavior, saying no to her stepmother. At the stage of discussion, the affect was only beginning to be active, so she needed to go deeper into the experience. I suggested the homework assignment of using a spiral-bound notebook to write her inner "truth with feeling" on the left side of the book and her contemporary and disconfirming wisdom on the right side. The moving result was quoted in Chapter 10. By suggesting that, I empowered her to do some of the memory reconsolidation work on her own. We reviewed her progress in the next session.

Having a universal framework means that knowledge from many sources can be assimilated, one lesson at a time, with what we already know. As we acquire more knowledge, we can use it to deepen and broaden our understanding of how humans heal and grow and what we can do to facilitate the processes that lead to improved lives.

Making use of our Rosetta Stone, we can now look at psychotherapy as a large collection of techniques and conceptualizations, ripe for rational mixing and matching to accomplish what needs to happen next in the client's voyage. This gives us a way of practicing psychotherapy integration while respecting and valuing the varied contributions of diverse therapies.

Key Points

- Two of the biggest incompatibilities between therapies are CBT's reluctance to talk about nonconscious information processing and PDT's relative prohibition against telling people what to do. It's time for them to meet in the middle.
- It is worth learning that science now exists to support the concept of nonconscious thought, and psychodynamic therapists have more than a one-hundred-year head start at learning to understand what's going on there.
- It is also worth noting that working with clients to support changes in behavior is one of the most powerful ways to send disconfirming messages (through experience) to the inner mind where they are needed.
- For other seemingly incompatible characteristics of different therapies, we apply a methodology of asking how each therapy supports the three clinical objectives required for change: new learning of improved coping responses, bringing affect into the room, and delivering disconfirming information to the inner mind in forms it can process.
- Therapies discussed include CBT, PDT, DBT, existential therapy, exposure therapy, ACT, EFT, EMDR, and IFS.
- Overall, the integrative framework we have built creates a kind of Rosetta Stone to help translate between diverse therapies to see that they all do the same few things in different ways.

REFERENCES

Beck, J. S. (2021). *Cognitive behavior therapy: Basics and beyond* (3rd ed.). Guilford Press.

Brenner, E., Schwartz, R., & Becker, C. (2023). Development of the internal family systems model: Honoring contributions from family systems therapies. *Family process*.

Foa, E. B., Hembree, E. A., & Rothbaum, B. O. (2007). *Prolonged exposure therapy for PTSD: Emotional processing of traumatic experiences* (Therapist guide). Oxford University Press.

Gabbard, G. O. (2017). *Long-term psychodynamic psychotherapy: A basic text* (3rd ed.). American Psychiatric Publishing.

Greenberg, L. (2006). Emotion-focused therapy: A synopsis. *Journal of Contemporary Psychotherapy*, *36*, 87–93.

Hayes, S. (2016). Acceptance and commitment therapy, relational frame theory, and the third wave of behavioral and cognitive therapies - republished article. *Behavior Therapy*, *47*(6), 869–885.

Hayes, S., & Hofmann, S. (2018). Survival circuits and therapy: From automaticity to the conscious experience of fear and anxiety. *Current Opinion in Behavioral Sciences, 24*, 21–25.

Kwon, H., & Silva, E. (2020). Mapping the landscape of behavioral theories: Systematic literature review. *Journal of Planning Literature, 35*, 161–179.

Leeds, A. (2016). *A guide to the standard EMDR therapy protocols for clinicians, supervisors, and consultants*. Springer Publishing.

Linehan, M. M. (2015). *DBT skills training manual* (2nd ed.). The Guilford Press.

Vaverková, Z., Milton, A., & Merlo, E. (2020). Retrieval-dependent mechanisms affecting emotional memory persistence: Reconsolidation, extinction, and the space in between. *Frontiers in Behavioral Neuroscience, 14*, 56.

Yalom, I. D. (2009). *The gift of therapy: An open letter to a new generation of therapists and their patients* (1st ed.). Harper Perennial.

CHAPTER 14

The End of a Voyage and the Beginning of a New One

Approaching the end of our voyage together, let's review what we have learned. I'm building this summary mainly around the Five Key Questions to leave you with a guide you can take with you as your conversations progress. Some of the cases we will follow are more familiar and others are chosen to exemplify how the questions get to the heart of those elements that psychotherapy can change. I'm using boldface to highlight key words that relate to concepts discussed at length in earlier chapters.

SEEKING ACCURATE EMPATHY

If there is one formula to carry with you in helping clients trade their outdated responses for better ones, it is seeking **accurate empathy**, otherwise called **complex caring**, an ever deepening, emotionally engaged understanding. Let your **curiosity** be your guide as you pursue understanding, not to label, but to put yourself in the shoes of this other human. Strengthen your curiosity by paying attention to **what you don't know** and test your **working hypotheses** as you observe the unfolding action.

Simply following this formula will show your client that they are important to you as an individual. That will go a long way toward building a **positive alliance** and having some credibility in the bank to help the two of you work through errors, misunderstandings, and inevitable **ruptures**.

DOI: 10.4324/9781003619659-15

Question 1: What Is the EMP?

From the first few minutes of your relationship, you will be homing in on the source of pain, the **chief complaint**, that brought your client to therapy. That will serve as the first source of **motivation** and energy to move the therapy along. As you seek to understand the cause of this pain, it will lead you to the **inner mind**, that subcortical, survival-oriented, nonconscious information processing brain, inherited from other mammals, and the author of the **entrenched maladaptive patterns** psychotherapy is designed to treat.

You will begin to ask what outdated strategy the client's inner mind is doing its best to implement in order to stay safe. Whether inherited from millennia of evolution, invented earlier in development, or devised at a point of trauma, the solution to some serious challenge or problem is the source of an **outdated strategy** and the cause of the kinds of pain psychotherapy can treat.

And there may be **layers** of EMPs. The earliest is first and addresses an original challenge, but when the inner mind **predicts failure**, a new layer is created. We work with whichever layer is the most accessible or the most important to unravel. While EMPs exist in a vast range of different forms, there are a few recognizable types. **Resistance EMPs** are the more superficial ones, created on the spot to keep psychotherapy from disturbing the inner mind's survival circuits. Another very important group is made up of the EMPs that use (inappropriate) **shame, guilt, and even pride** to police their behavior. The key to those **judgment-based EMPs** is that they are based on internalized **values, attitudes, ideals, and prohibitions**. Those unhealthy standards are what need to change. They are heavily guarded against change and held particularly firmly. They are the basis of **internal critics** and the **inappropriate shame and guilt** they produce.

As we seek to clarify the presence and nature of EMPs, it will help to use **affect**, the bodily manifestation of nonconscious emotion, as our **North Star**, guiding the way to what is important. When affect is **in the room**, our job is to listen and learn its meaning, which automatically soothes the client and helps them be ready to heal and grow. When affect is **near but not quite there**, it's an opportunity to work with the client using empathic understanding to encourage access to feeling. Finally, affect may be **far away**, suppressed due to the action of hidden EMPs in the form of personality traits, judgment-based EMPs, and finely tuned habits. Only when these patterns change will relevant affect come into the room.

Here are examples. Let's follow them through each of the Five Key Questions.

Question 1: Examples

Margaret, age 60 years, has an EMP demanding that she squash herself down to a size her father could tolerate, so she would not be banished from the family she needed for survival. In a second layer of EMP, an internal critic comes to reinforce the prohibition against being visible and uses intense shame as a deterrent. This leaves her with the chief complaint of an adult life that has been dull and undistinguished.

Mark, age 38 years, suffers from an EMP requiring him to compete and win out over everyone else to find and keep the love he has needed to make his way in life. In adulthood, he must always be competing and vigilant, lest someone else appear with more attractive qualities to dazzle and take away his wife's affection. The resulting stress is often overwhelming. It makes him angry to see others who don't have to work so hard and yet seem happy.

Lorraine, age 68 years, has a deep fear that death will come too soon, and she will never have the life she wanted. Her inner mind produces anxiety, probably enhanced genetically, and her EMP is that her inner mind projects metaphors into consciousness to express her anxiety. Her consciousness takes these literally and puts hope in worrying about medical complications that could possibly happen, and what to do about them. These take all her energy and make her even more anxious, yet fail to make her ready for the many real-life dangers that might come from any direction and without warning.

Fiona, a student, age 20 years, introduced in Chapter 5, was ready as a child to do anything for love, which was scarce. Her EMP strategy was built on the idea that the way to attract it was to achieve great skill in art. She was sure there was no other way to gain love, but her strategy was failing, and she was losing hope. The harder she tried, the more deeply she fell into despair.

Harold, age 75 years, learned early in life from his chaotic family that he could not count on anyone. They were well-meaning, but not up to the job. His main EMP strategy was to trust only himself, but that was too lonely, and he also held a desperate and shameful hope that if he were clever enough, someone might notice and come to his rescue. After a lifetime of striving and waiting, he was still going back and forth between half-hearted, ineffective attempts to find reliable caring and turning away to trust only himself.

Each of these plans was full of hope but going nowhere. Each was constructed with desperation and care. Each was fiercely guarded but doomed to fail. Each of the protagonists needed someone with knowledge of the sea and of boats, and possessing a reliable compass.

Question 2: The DREAD

The only way the inner mind/brain is able to tag threats is by a neural activation or **warning signal** consisting of **nonconscious emotion**. That is the inner **DREAD** that EMPs seek to suppress. The **inner mind** has many **survival circuits**. Each one takes in information from the environment, from memory, and from within and applies the first schema, the **threat detection schema**, to predict if a threat is near. If so, it produces the **warning signal/nonconscious emotion** that triggers a second, **response selection schema** which launches a response, starting with affects and conscious thoughts and feelings that tell us the nature of what is **DREADED**. When we notice affect and learn about the nature of the **DREAD**, it helps us develop an understanding and accurate empathy about just what it is the inner mind is dreading, that is, what is the threat the inner mind is responding to.

Margaret was dreading being banished from her family (of origin), and, through a second EMP, dreading the sense of shame that would accompany any attempt to make herself noticed in the world.

Mark was dreading the possibility of having his bit of love stolen away, leaving him alone and empty.

Lorraine was dreading that she might die alone.

Fiona was dreading coming to a final failure in her search for love.

Harold is still dreading the ultimate emergency, and his inner mind is still wasting energy and life trying to be braced and ready for it.

Question 3: Your THEORY

With the beginnings of answers to the first two questions, we have the makings of a hypothesis about how and possibly why the client's EMP was created. It represents a **strategy** for suppressing or eliminating the dreaded **nonconscious emotion**, which functions as a **proxy** for a serious threat or challenge. The inner mind makes rapid approximations, using predictive coding, to **pattern match** with past experience, predict a threat, and launch a response as quickly as possible.

Here is where we try to understand the **first author** of the EMP. We can think of it as simply a response, but the inner mind functions more like an **inner self**. Much like other mammals, we have a basic, survival-oriented brain, the subcortical, limbic, inner mind with its survival circuits. That is where EMPs originate. Frozen in time and cut off from the rest of the mind, the **EMP** operates like an inner self in the sense that it has a **strategy**, a **plan**, and **hope** for success, which energize the **motivation** to carry it out, along with ways to follow the likelihood of success and how close or far it may be. That self can bear characteristics of a level of **development** that identify its origins as well as suggesting, in the light of the client's life history, what the original threat might have been.

This is only a **theory**, and it may take on more detail and change as the therapy progresses, so we remember to hold it with a **light touch**. A theory is a prediction. It is an attempt to explain what we observe. As such, it also invites being **tested**. This is where the continuing flow of new information and progress in therapy can serve tentatively as confirmations that we are or are not on the right track.

Margaret's trouble started with fear of her father's biting criticism when he came home drunk. Her first EMP was to squash herself to avoid banishment, but her natural spunkiness threatened to make her talk back. The threat that her first EMP would ultimately fail triggered the formation of a second layer of EMP, a set of values that attracting attention was shameful. An **inner critic** came to the rescue, shaming her out of her ambitions and wishes to be noticed. From then on, she lived a life of excessive modesty and had only occasional fantasies of writing violent novels to express her inner self's true feelings. The trigger for her shame was any thought or action suggesting that she had value.

Mark's experience as a schoolboy told him it was the accomplishments and attributes of popular kids that brought them the attention and love he had never received. His EMP was to focus on his performance, hoping to win the contest for success and attractiveness, while constantly doubting his success. Fear and anger were set off whenever he underperformed or doubted his prowess. He had never experienced someone like the wife he married well into adulthood, who was simply attached to him. He interpreted her actions according to his inner schemas. His adult trigger was that whenever he doubted himself, he would doubt her and think she didn't really love him. Then he felt angry and cheated that his hard work had not been appreciated.

Lorraine's fear was deep and partly genetic. Her inner mind carried the feeling that disaster could strike at any moment. Her EMP was to generate automatic thoughts as metaphors for this inner dread. Her conscious mind further amplified their frightening quality with semi-realistic scenarios to reinforce the need to spend all her energy worrying.

Perhaps that would help her be prepared. That was her inner mind's strategy.

Fiona's early life failure to find love from her family led to her developing an erroneous theory that performance must be the way to their hearts. It didn't work, but she assumed that was because her skill was still not perfect. Despair and depression came from repeatedly giving her all, with no success.

Harold's family was chaotic, and when he was five, his father ragefully threatened to abandon the family. He saw that his parents were not up to the job in any real emergency, so he hung his hope on becoming capable of handling anything. He also held onto a small hope that extraordinary abilities might endear him to his mother or, later, some substitute. He vacillated between those two sources of hope but didn't commit fully to either one.

Question 4: The RESPONSE

The **second, response selection schema**, uses predictive coding to determine the details of the EMP. With this question, we look at what might be a better answer, a **more satisfactory RESPONSE**. What is maladaptive about the existing pattern of response? Is there a better way? Does the new response have to be built from scratch, or can it be adapted from another one in the client's previous experience? Sometimes the healthy response is to recognize that what was once a threat is no longer. In that case, there is no need for an alternative response, only the possibility of changing the **threat detection schema** to indicate no threat.

Improved responses become available through **new learning** in a way similar to sports moves. But learning from scratch is a big investment. It is usually more efficient and effective for clients to adapt an existing response pattern than to learn an entirely new one. Any form of success can supply the makings of a new and improved approach to a problem. The most common adult alternative to EMPs developed in childhood is **acceptance**. That's because children hold so tightly to hope and seem to be programmed not to let it go. Acceptance means making peace with the fact that parents are dysfunctional or that bad things can happen but can't be fully anticipated. The result is a transformation from the constant angst of trying to eliminate a threat to a peaceful readiness to handle whatever comes.

Margaret's fear of banishment from the family has teamed up with her dreaded inner critic to deter her from any attempt to find interest or brilliance in her life. Transformative change helped rewrite her dread of banishment, but the inner critic is a tougher adversary and continues to give out inappropriate shame. That will require following new patterns of civil disobedience. For her, that means saying no to her stepmother and putting herself in a position to be noticed. Success in these actions puts pressure on her inner critic to recognize that values favoring false modesty are unnecessary and wrong.

Mark has exhausted himself in competing but has little experience with trusting and counting on his partner's attachment. Acting as if she can be trusted to care about him will be a new experience for him, but not too difficult to learn. That will deliver disconfirming information to his inner self, that her attachment does not depend on his performance. Early attempts at trusting will be helped by his wife and him working together at being good to each other and not taking their relationship for granted.

Lorraine's tendency to fearfulness is probably inborn and there to stay, but she can teach herself to be at peace with it by being fully aware that it is a natural predisposition and has nothing to do with the true level of risk in her life. Furthermore, there are only very limited things adults can do to ensure their safety and freedom from health surprises. Learning to accept and tolerate internal anxiety can be a learned skill, which, over time, is generally superior to continually seeking reassurance.

Fiona achieved remarkable skill but no love. She will need to practice asking for love instead of trying to earn it. Positive results will help her add new confidence and experience to her considerable, but formerly unrecognized, interpersonal strengths.

Harold became extraordinarily self-sufficient but felt no safer. Letting go of protections is hard to do, as self-protectiveness of this kind is so automatic. He will need to gain experience with being vulnerable as well as acting with conviction in asking more from others.

Question 5: The ANTIDOTE

This new information serves two functions. By **colliding** with the old "truth" it sets the old **implicit learning** of schemas into a **volatile** state, meaning that the old predictive coding is now subject to being **re-written**. The second function of this disconfirming information is to provide the **content** for rewriting schemas using **memory reconsolidation**. It will dictate the new **response** pattern to be selected when triggered by the same inputs as before.

As indicated above, there are two schemas, potentially to be changed. One is information to show that the threatening circumstance no longer warrants a response, and the other is to modify what response to select.

These correspond to the two schemas that once initiated the client's EMP, the **threat detection schema** and the **response selection schema**.

Most importantly, the art of psychotherapy is making sure the **ANTIDOTE** is delivered to the subcortical structures where the **schemas** and their **implicit learning** reside as **procedural memory**. **Experiential information** is nonverbal already, and, as such, is easily delivered where it is needed. Other information, such as ideas, must be translated into nonverbal, associative forms as it makes its way down to the **subcortical brain**.

Margaret experienced transformative change when she said out loud that her **DREAD** was being banished from her family of origin. Simply articulating this "truth" was the main thing that awoke the conscious realization that her family of origin no longer exists, while her husband is highly satisfactory and unlikely to banish her. With the **communication channel** wide open, as indicated by tears, her new realization was transformative. On the other hand, it left an **inner critic**, adhering to false values and continuing to cause inappropriate shame. The antidote for that is civil disobedience, leading to successful and pleasurable experiences of being noticed.

Mark needed to realize that his wife's love is not transactional, that she is firmly attached to him, and that makes her want to stay and find closeness with him. This was complicated and was not easily deliverable to the **subcortical brain**. He needs to focus on experiences when he sensed her attachment even though his dysfunctional mistrust had made him treat her as untrustworthy.

Lorraine was afraid of dying alone. The **antidote** for her was **accepting** that she would one day die, and that worrying or bracing for it would not improve the experience. Once again, this is not an easy antidote to **deliver**. The idea that death might not be so terrible is a **negative,** and those do not **compute** in the subcortical inner mind. The best for her is constructing her own image of dying peacefully, surrounded by loving family members. Forming the image of that experience was possible but was made harder by the premature and distressing death of her own mother, from whom she had never received much love.

Fiona had almost completely lost hope and had gone into a profound depression in which her **SEEKING** system was at a low ebb. She needed to dare to contact former friends despite the risk of rejection. Fortunately (through positive regard by her therapists), she was unusually expressive of her needs and receptive to receiving appreciation from others. She took the risk several times, and in each instance was quite successful. That began to lift her out of the depression. That energized her

SEEKING system to provide energy for her to repeat the positive experience. She was on her way.

Harold was **braced** against the ultimate emergency, so he had trouble taking in the support of those around him. He needed the experience of true support during a particularly difficult time when his wife freely gave it. That experience got through to his inner mind and helped contradict his mistrust, but only at a medium level. He still had trouble in the form of an isolating response when he felt most vulnerable. The **working hypothesis** is now that this partial result was limited due to having internalized a **value** that said he did not deserve to be supported, and therefore accepting support would cause a **dreaded** dose of **shame**.

WE ARE NAVIGATORS

Just as seafarers need a navigator who knows the charts and the waters, our clients need us to be navigators to guide them on a scary and tumultuous journey to somewhere unknown. In this book and this chapter's summary, I have tried to show some waypoints for your own journey. In doing so, I have tried to lay out the basic elements that will guide you and your clients through storms and the unexpected. It is my sincere hope that our trip together will help you be more ready than ever to be a confident navigator, prepared to help your clients on their own exciting and scary but ultimately safe passages.

Key Points

- In this last chapter, we use the five key questions to follow five cases as they unfold. In so doing, we develop a kind of summary of the framework that describes the infrastructure of all therapies.
- In the end, we hope to help therapists view our profession as one treatment with many fine techniques and conceptualizations to draw from as we navigate. By knowing what we want them to do and how they work, we are no longer hampered by concerns about incompatibility or lack of fidelity to a specific formula.

Appendix: Biology Meets Psychology—Some Notes

This is an appendix because, while needed, it is informal and consists of personal impressions, rather than solidly grounded conclusions. I am not proposing a way of thinking about therapy or how that framework influences practice. Instead, issues around biological factors come up so often and have such a real influence on psychotherapy that I decided to share what follows, mainly from my own experience. I am offering these notes, based mainly on five decades of observation and learning. These should not be considered definitive but may represent helpful starting points. They are, in many cases, my working hypotheses, to be held lightly, as they may change with further observation and knowledge.

In some cases, biology is the predominant causative factor. In others, the basic problem is psychological, but biology becomes a relevant factor.

BIOLOGY AS A CAUSATIVE FACTOR

There is little question that biological factors primarily cause several serious mental problems. Here, I emphasize the ways that biology appears to have an impact on psychological/emotional functioning, which, then, can be the focus of psychotherapy.

BIPOLAR ILLNESS

To my observation, bipolar illness is one of the most biological of psychiatric problems. While episodes appear to be triggered by life events, it also happens that subtle beginnings of an episode influence responses to events. What looks in retrospect like a response, may be better explained as a relapse of the illness leading to some form of conflict with the outside world. The difference may not change the approach to therapy, but it seems wise to be aware of the two possibilities. Bipolar illness is one place where the medical model discussed in Chapter 5 largely does apply. Pharmacological treatment for each phase, whether dominated by depression, irritability, or some degree of mania, is moderately effective. So far, no medication seems to guarantee freedom from relapse. To make things more complex, some people have continuous high energy but not episodes of depression or mania. In those cases, it is the client's quality of life that determines whether to intervene. There are also people without mania, whose depression appears biological and responds better to antipsychotic and mood stabilizing medicaton than to antidepressants. I tend to think of them as "having bipolar depression."

Psychotherapy may help with maladaptive responses to the biology, but it does not appear to change the underlying illness. The exception is that denial of illness often leads to refusal of medication and a worse outcome. In cases of extreme denial, helpers may be in the terrible position of waiting for a bad situation to become worse so that societal policies can allow hospitalization. In such cases, the goal of therapy may be acceptance of the illness and the need for treatment. An educated and accepting client can often reverse an early relapse of either kind by taking medication immediately at the onset of an episode. Especially those who do not deny their illness can and do lead productive and satisfying lives.

DEPRESSION

People can become profoundly depressed for purely psychological reasons, as in the case of Fiona, or for purely biological reasons as well as anything in between. The biological ones tend to suffer more from feeling much worse in the early morning, from early morning waking, and rapid weight loss. The more purely psychological ones tend to have fewer biological signs and to have clear reasons for emotional despair. Clear doesn't always mean obvious. It could be the failure of a secret goal or a moral principle. Even when I think the initial cause is psychological, some people have a predisposition and start at some point to slip into the symptoms listed above for the biological kind of depression. I think of that as a vicious cycle that gets started in the mind, then triggers a reaction in the body. In those cases, I go ahead with medication as well as talk.

Fiona's depression was caused when childlike failed attempts to find love and relationships continued into young adulthood, still with no success. Her despair was approaching a crescendo with active suicidal thoughts. An attempt to remove her depressive symptoms without addressing the cause would have caused even greater despair. Appropriate work with the psychological issues led to recovery.

On the other hand, Ethan, an older adult man presented with a year of glum feelings after retiring. After a year, he began to experience weight loss and feeling terrible in the early morning. It looked like a biological vicious cycle had gradually gotten started. He responded rapidly to medication and subsequently showed no indications of emotional pathology.

The lesson is that these are not easy determinations and depend on psychiatric judgment, as well as some trial and error. The literature offers some statistical help.

ANXIETY

Susceptibility to anxiety runs in families and most of the time, has a strong genetic and biological component. The way I conceptualize it, the inner mind is prone to perceiving the world as highly dangerous. It then projects into consciousness metaphors to capture the way it feels. These appear as phobias and specific disaster scenarios. Clients tend to amplify these (catastrophize) with ideas of dire future consequences. The end results are anxiety and panic attacks that can fuel themselves in a vicious cycle. Chasing relief by seeking outside reassurance only makes the anxiety worse. Understanding where scary thoughts come from is helpful in taking the focus away from trying to deal with them as if they were the actual problem. In many cases the best long-term outcome may be when the individual stops seeking complete relief and accepts that some anxiety is part of life.

OCD

Obsessive-compulsive problems range from mild symptoms to full-blown rituals and intrusive thoughts. They seem to act like anxiety in that they are based on a biological tendency, which is not very susceptible to psychological treatment. What does work is response prevention therapy, where, as in exposure therapy, the client voluntarily faces the anxiety, which becomes intense when they refrain from performing rituals. By making anxiety tolerable, the impact of OCD on life is lessened. The equivalent for obsessive thoughts, in contrast to performing ritual acts, is letting them play and not doing anything to try to eliminate them. The result is increased ability to accept anxiety and a better life.

PANIC

According to Panksepp, panic comes from a different system, the one that responds to a built-in fear of aloneness. In contrast to anxiety and OCD, I think there often is a psychological basis. When panic attacks happen, I believe first that the inner mind has encountered something in life that it considers highly dangerous and that events are re-triggering some traumatic memory or experience. Finding and treating the underlying psychological issue is often successful. After a panic attack, fear of having another one adds significantly to the impact. That's why any measures to suppress the next attack can help move the client into a calmer, less anxious state. The alternative to bottom-up treatment is accepting the attacks and learning to live with them or using as-needed medication for occasional ones. This can sometimes be more successful than trying to eliminate them entirely. SSRI antidepressants do suppress panic attacks fairly effectively but have the disadvantage of later withdrawal producing the opposite effect from their benefit: abnormally heightened emotionality, which can last for months.

SCHIZOPHRENIA

While medication is the mainstay of treatment, I am intrigued by the fact that many of the symptoms seem to involve a fragility of the sense of self-integrity, meaning where the self ends and the outside world begins. Symptoms often involve fear of separation as well as irrational ideas of influence from outside. A classic prelude to relapse is the primitive logic of trying to become more independent by stopping treatment, which then leads to symptomatic relapse. The developmental era represented by such symptoms appears to go back to very early, pre-one-year-old development. Does that mean development was faulty from the beginning? Or that the biology of the illness causes regression in the client's developmental level? I don't know. There is room for psychotherapeutic work on those issues with the goal of increasing learned skills and resilience.

ADDICTION

I think of addiction as ranging from highly biological in origin to mostly psychological. In either case, we see an inner mind convinced that survival requires using the substance. Even when the conscious mind wants to be sober, the ways the inner mind has of influencing behavior show not only its power but also the broad range of tools the subcortical inner mind uses to control voluntary choices. These range from rationalizations to distractions, to impulses, and even subtle strategies like the principle of one thing leads to another, where the conscious self is tricked into making a seemingly benign choice that predictably and eventually leads to relapse. In this way, the inner mind's survival tools become the factors that maintain the illness despite terrible costs.

In my mind, the most powerful treatment is pitting one biological force against another. The core of AA is human connection. That is a biological need at the same level of power as the compulsion to use the substance as a means of survival. That way, AA counters the need for the substance with the need for human connection. Besides that, motivational interviewing does have an excellent toolbox for dealing with denial and a highly reactive inner self, intent on maintaining the status quo.

While medications have been shown to reduce relapse rates by a percentage, I remain concerned that they send a false message to the inner mind that the hard work of accessing recovery-oriented activities is not needed. Clients often feel as if medication will work without great effort on their part. This encourages false hope in the medical model. The recovery model is more appropriate, and those who are successful tend to be the ones who are unconditionally committed to recovery and hungry for it.

ADHD

The primary symptoms of ADHD affect about 5 percent of the population and make these individuals feel different from peers. They crave intensity and struggle to focus without it. That's why they write school papers the night before they are due. When their interest is engaged, they tend to be hyper-focused and can be highly effective, but task switching is hard and generates irritation. Dread of getting into the next task may be the driver of procrastination. Limited working memory leads them to make obvious mistakes and requires significant compensation to succeed in detail work. They are impulsive, as well as spontaneous and creative, and may not see distant consequences until they are imminent. This relative insensitivity to eventual consequences may increase susceptibility to addictions.

A prominent psychological effect is low self-esteem resulting from frequent poor performance in tasks designed for 95 percent of the population. This is particularly true during school years. Psychotherapy helps with this. It can also help clients accept their neurodiversity and find niches where they fit best.

Medication helps increase focus on boring tasks such as schoolwork, scheduling, and organization. School is inherently biased against ADHD people in that it emphasizes organization and planning. Following the school years, routine tasks are better avoided or delegated, but when necessary, they can be aided with drug treatment. The most important principle is that it is okay to shape life around the individual's strengths and interests, rather than the client trying (vainly) to be like the 95 percent.

AUTISM

My experience is with high-functioning autism clients. They do best when they are aware and accepting of their neurodiversity. Then they can use resources and guidance to learn rules of behavior that help them function in the world. They can find niches that take advantage of memory capacity and reduced sensitivity to situations that give others trouble. One client was open to the idea of being an embalmer because dead bodies didn't bother him.

Reduced sensitivity to social cues means that therapists who are used to the relationship being a major tool for positive influence need to remember that the basis for their being helpful will likely not be the same.

Index

acceptance 108, 149–150; and commitment therapy 188
accurate empathy 16–17, 100, 127
adaptations 22
advertisers 137
affects 18, 43, 62, 83, 126
Alan 132
Alexander & French 111
amygdala 88
antidote 108
anxiety 41
art of psychotherapy 137–138
associative thinking 89
attachment 32
attitudes 77
authenticity 138
automatic thoughts 63, 83
avoidance 129

backlash 144, 148
basic trust 60
Beck, Judith 184
biases 140–141
Biven, Lucy 55
bodily responses 85
boundaries 174
brain networks 127
breathing 44

Carole 146, 148, 169, 181
central executive network 128
civil disobedience 79, 144, 148
closure 150
cognitive behavioral therapy 179
common factors 14–16, 133
communication channel 57–58, 104
complex caring 17, 128
Conan, Vivian 141
conscience 77–79
consequences 87
countertransference 68, 81
culture 174
curiosity 11–12

default mode network 128
deprivation 79–80
development 118–119, 161–162
dialectical behavior therapy 177, 185–186
DiClemente, C. 143
dissociative identity disorder 61, 141
dopamine 154
dread 104–106

Ecker, Bruce 21, 122, 144
Ellen 12

emotion 22, 56; focused therapy 47, 189; in-session 56, 101; nonconscious 83
Entrenched Maladaptive Patterns (EMP) 28, 96–98; strategies 96–98
epigenetics 62, 115
Evans, Joseph 59
evolution 23, 123
existential therapy 186–187
experience 143–144
exposure therapy 121, 187–188
extinction 114, 121
Eye Movement Desensitization and Reprocessing (EMDR) 132, 189–190

feelings 63–64, 83
Fiona 197
five key questions 100
flow of information 21
Foa, Edna 121
formulation 13
Freud, Sigmund 67

Gabbard, Glen 68
George 42
guilt 77

Harold 200
Hayes, Steven 31

ideals 77
implicit 26
impulses 64, 83
incompatibilities 182
information 21, 108, 120, 122; disconfirming 108, 122; encoding of 120
informed consent 144
infrastructure 15, 21
inner critic 77, 148
inner mind 22, 25
instrumental emotions 47
intellect 127–128
internal family systems therapy 190–191
internalized standards 77

John 39, 117

Kahneman, Daniel 59
Kandel, Eric 90, 120
kill the messenger 95–96

labeling 13, 100
learned fear response 87
Ledoux, Joseph 31, 55
Levine, Peter 163
logic nonconscious 90–91
Lorraine 197

manipulation 138–139
Margaret 93, 129, 147–148, 192, 197
Maria 69
Mark 197
medical model 71
memory reconsolidation 18, 29–30, 114, 121–122
metacommunication 48
Miller 138
mind 21
mindfulness 18, 44, 47
misattribution 139
moments of meaning 133
moral weight 172
motivation 85, 153
motivational interviewing 138, 164

Nader, Karim 122
Nancy 15, 145, 156
negative feedback loop 96
neutrality 169
new learning 107–108, 114
(ninteen sixties)1960s 173
nonconscious emotion 88
nonlinear 91

outdated responses 27
outside influences 164
Oxnam, Robert 61–62

panic attacks 39
Panksepp, Jaak 55, 88, 154

pattern recognition 84
personal therapy 175
personification 54–55
pitfalls 176
planning 73–74
poetry 89–90
prediction error 91, 108, 122
predictive coding 84
procedural memory 84
process 67
Prochaska, J. 143
prohibitions 77
psychodynamic therapy 179

question 45

reactance 138
recovery model 72–73
repertoire 107
resistance 35, 145
response prevention therapy 121
response selection schema 83, 88–89, 92, 107, 147
Rogers, Carl 17
Rosetta Stone 191–192
rule 107
rupture 81, 140

schemas 139
Schwartz, Richard 54–55
SEEKING system 154–155
shame and guilt 77–78, 165
sleep 122
Smith, Jeffrey 122
somatic experiencing therapy 163
spiral bound book 79, 148
stages of change 143
story 104
subcortical 25
subunits of pathology 20, 28
supervision 100
support 175–176
survival circuits 91–93
symptom resolution 67
system 1 26

theory 13, 106–107
thinking fast 26
thinking slow 86
Thomas 80
threat detection schema 83, 88–89, 108–110, 147
threat processing 130
three clinical objectives 182
three step dance 47–49
top-down change 86
Tournier, Paul 10
transference 74
transformative change 100
trauma bonds 140
trust 16

values 27, 77, 144, 148–149
Victorian era 173

Wampold, B. 14
warning signal 83, 88, 93–95, 104
working hypothesis 13–14

For Product Safety Concerns and Information please contact our EU
representative GPSR@taylorandfrancis.com
Taylor & Francis Verlag GmbH, Kaufingerstraße 24, 80331 München, Germany

www.ingramcontent.com/pod-product-compliance
Ingram Content Group UK Ltd.
Pitfield, Milton Keynes, MK11 3LW, UK
UKHW022352190926
475702UK00015B/2255

* 9 7 8 1 0 4 1 0 2 5 1 6 0 *